15Minute.Fitness Fat Loss Formula

Workout Smarter Not Harder!

The Easy Way to Lose Weight, Tone Up and Build Lean Muscle for Life

Jonas Schwartz, PhD(cand.), MA, M.Hum, MBA

Jackie Schwartz, BA Exercise Science, CPT

JONAS & JACKIE SCHWARTZ

DEDICATION

This work is dedicated first and foremost to my Creator and Redeemer and Sanctifier. I can never be worthy of such benevolence—only grateful. And that I am.

Second only to God, this is dedicated to my Angel, Jackie Schwartz. God knew I needed you, and I never would have seen sharing healthy living as a ministry had you not opened my eyes.

Next, this work is dedicated to my six children and eleven grandchildren. I look forward to future editions which allow me to amend this number (of grandchildren!)

Finally, this work is dedicated to normal people with real lives and families. I speak to you—not to elite athletes, but to those who need the easiest, most efficient and most effective way to health, strength and leanness. You CAN work out for hours, starve yourself and turn your whole life upside down. But you don't HAVE to. There is a better way—for you and for your children after you...

CONTENTS

INTRODUCTION:

WELCOME!

If you bought a copy of this book, then I would highly encourage you to visit www.15minute.fitness and enroll in our Free Foundation course. It uses short videos to give a high-level overview of the terrain we will cover in depth here in this book. It will also give you 30 day access to my free beginner's workout program on the training app we use with our paid clients.

Just go to www.15minute.fitness and sign up for our "Free Foundations Course." It is a one page course with five short lessons that explain our basic approach. At the end of that page, you'll find links to a free meal plan and sample workout. You will also be automatically enrolled in a free month of our 15Minute.Fitness workout app.

Too many people fail in their health and fitness pursuits due to lack of preparation. Taking the little time necessary to lay solid foundations makes all the difference. Our clients who have followed that one page course have shown exponentially better results than those who choose not to.

OUR STORIES

Finding "ME" Again
(Jackie Schwartz)

I was never skinny as a kid. I wasn't fat but "solid" was often used to describe my build. In college, I loved the aerobics craze and worked out a lot. I found that my solid build was strong and I enjoyed lifting weights. I enjoyed it so much that I majored in Exercise Science. I looked great but not as good as the "skinny" girls around me - I was still more "solid". It was hard being a "thick" aerobics instructor—so hard that I turned to unhealthy practices and developed an eating disorder. I battled for a while with anorexia and bulimia, a cycle that wreaked havoc on my metabolism. After counseling, I vowed to take better care of my body, and healthy, nutritional food became important.

When I married, I weighed 145 pounds. I was in my BMI. I considered it my "happy weight", meaning I didn't kill myself working out. I just took a daily walk and ate healthy enough, still enjoying dinners out, wine and treats now and then. When I had my kids, I was able to return to, and maintain, that 145 pound "happy weight". As I neared 40, several things happened. My hormones started to change. Weight crept on, slowly at first. My marriage was deteriorating. I wasn't paying attention to my weight or my health. I was too worried about everything else around me.

At 42, I could not save my marriage, and when I was forced to look at myself in pictures, I did not even recognize the person I saw anymore. I was embarrassed at how much weight I had put on. My weight had reached 185. Finding pictures at that weight is hard, because I avoided the camera like the plague. I avoided activities with my kids that involved shorts or a bathing suit. That summer, the doctor told me that my cholesterol was high and that I was borderline diabetic.

I knew I had to make changes—I was 40 pounds heavier than I was all of my adult life. And now I was single, and my boys were going to need me to BE THERE for them now more than ever. It was a traumatic time for them too, and I needed to be in a healthy place to support them. I knew how to eat healthy—I used to eat that way. I used to cook healthy family meals, not just rely on take out. I used to move more playing with the kids—not just veg out in front of the TV giving into depression. I felt guilty and realized what a bad example I had set for them the last few years. So, I took action.

I cleaned up my diet. I went back to eating "healthy enough", still enjoying dinners out, treats and wine. I also started walking again—nothing big, just a 25 to 30 minute walk about five days a week. The first summer at the doc was great. I had lost 20 pounds and the doc was happy. Moving from teaching in the classroom to teaching PE helped my activity level. But I got stuck at 150. I wanted so badly to be back at 145 and hear the doc say that I am in the healthy BMI range. I could not make it happen. I even joined a gym and started lifting weights again.

Then I met Jonas. At first, I gained a few pounds when we started dating. Dating was fun and we splurged a lot!! But it did not take long for me to decide I had to reign it back in. It was easy. I had a partner who had the same healthy goals in mind that I had. Jonas loved everything I cooked and was often shocked at the nutritional counts of our supper. He even enjoyed the healthy meals I packed for lunch so much that he asked me to prep some for him as well. I had hoped my weight-lifting workouts at the gym would get me to my goal, but it wasn't working. Jonas offered to create a program for me and be my coach. He told me he wanted me to give up my hour-long sessions several times a week for just 15 minutes a day.

I thought he was crazy. I wasn't sure I believed him when he told me that he only worked out 15 minutes a day. But I did it. And within weeks, I could see changes in my body. My muscles were suddenly responding to my workouts. I was getting stronger and at the same time getting leaner. While writing this, I now weigh137 pounds. And last week my athlete son had to admit that I won our summer ab challenge.

I have no more issues doing activities with my children in a bathing suit. I can keep up with them, and my confidence is almost as high as my energy. I love knowing I am feeding my family quality food, still treating them (I LOVE to bake!) and showing them a healthy balance that they can carry on into their adult life. Being a parent isn't easy, knowing you are setting the foundation for your child's future is scary. The least I can do is try my best to set a healthy foundation!

—Jackie Nors Schwartz

Unlovable
(Jonas Schwartz)

I was a fat kid. Actually, in pretty much every class I was in through Junior High, I was THE fat kid. My granny raised me, and she fed me well—really well. She was loving her adopted son the best she knew how, but as my body grew fatter and fatter, I grew more and more miserable and isolated inside.

When I was 12 or 13, what I wanted most in the world was a girlfriend. I had a crush on a girl for years. But the last person any girl wanted was the fat nerd in school. I felt unlovable.

I remember sitting at home alone at night wishing I could take a knife and cut off my belly. I visualized the whole process. I would be free of that hateful burden. I would no longer be unlovable. Then someone could love me.

Puberty kicked in and I got a surge of motivation. I played volleyball, soccer, jogged and starved away a full 60 pounds by the time I was 15. That was amazing! I remember showing a friend on my volleyball team a photo of me when I was young and fat. He said, "Look! It's the kid who ate Schwartz!" LOL.

And then at age 35, I hit a wall. I had moved to Ennis Texas (south of Dallas) to take care of my Dad who had been diagnosed with ALS (Lou Gehrig's Disease). I moved in with him and my stepmom (who has gold, saint's wings waiting on her). I stayed home with him and helped however I could.

But, my magical youthful hormones had declined to aging levels, I couldn't devote hours to sports anymore, and I began putting weight back on. Within two years, I'd gained those 60 pounds back again, plus another 20.

I remember every time I would look in the mirror, I would think, "That's not ME." And I would hear my friend's voice in my ear saying, "Look, it's the guy who ate Schwartz!" I started feeling like I did when I was a young boy—alone and unlovable. Depression kicked in.

Around this time, my first grandson was born. I imagined all the wonderful things that we would be able to do together. I had not grown up living with my own father, so this was a chance to experience a side of life I had not personally known. I was going to make it count! I wanted him to know and love his Granddad.

Shortly after he was born, I remember sitting on my couch, putting on my shoes. Merely bending over to tie my laces turned into a traumatic event. I remember straining hard, all the blood rushing to my face, turning it bright red. When I was able to sit back up, my head was swimming. I was dizzy and seeing stars.

I don't know exactly what happened to me while trying to tie my shoes that day, but it was then I knew that my dreams of doing cool stuff with my new grandson were just silly fantasies. How was I going to teach him how to throw a football or how to ride a bike if I was in such bad shape that I couldn't even bend over to tie my shoes?

I knew, if I wanted to live much longer, if I wanted to play with my grandson, if I wanted him to actually know his granddad, I had to make my own health a priority in my life. One of the fathers of the church in a book called the Didache says there are two roads open before us, one leads to death, and one leads to life. I chose life.

I was older now, and I didn't have the energy I had as a kid, when I ran off that 60 pounds of baby fat. Plus, I had a job and a family. I couldn't give up hours out of my day to get this done. There were not enough hours in the day as it was. I knew I had work smarter, not harder. I had become a college professor, and so I did what I had been educated to do. I began researching.

If you've ever begun researching dieting and exercise, you know there is a ton of information out there, and one article conflicts with the next. There are a lot of "maps" on how to get out of those deep, dark woods of ill-health, but they say conflicting things. Logic says they can't ALL be right.

Luckily, I partnered with an enormously competent coach who did more than give me a map. He acted as my guide and got me out of those woods with scientifically verifiable principles tailored and applied to my particular situation. He filtered the signal from the noise, distilled the concepts into action steps, and showed me how to implement them within the parameters of my own particular personal life situation. That, my brothers and sisters, is priceless.

It took me a solid year of steady progress, but I lost the 60 pounds of fat and started gaining muscle. I'm not trying to win any powerlifting competitions, but having more muscle lets me eat more food and not get fat. And I like to eat! It really is the secret to fighting the hormonal decline as we age. I felt better. I had more energy. I had more confidence. I was treated differently. I saw ME in the mirror again, and for the first time, it was a positive, not a negative. At the time of this writing, I am 47 years old, and I am honestly in the best shape of my life—by far!

There is a reason for all the positive energy and emotion that comes with bodily health. Humans are not disembodied spirits. We are unities of body and soul. In my faith, our spirit is our intellect and identity, and our bodies are our channels of activity, as well as our very first gift from God. When either is sick, corrupt, or out of balance, we are not whole as we were made to be. And, I believe I will be called to account on how I cared for this fundamental gift. I want to hear, "Well done, my good and faithful servant. Since you were faithful in small matters, I will give you great responsibilities. Come, share your master's joy." (Mt 25:23).

I want that for other people too. If you can relate to that sad, lonely fat kid, or that aging man who no longer felt like "ME", then I want to help you. I now play with all my grandkids at the park and on the waterslides (yeah, I'm THAT guy), and you know what? I wouldn't trade that for the world. God bless you. Thanks for listening. Now, choose life.

—Jonas Schwartz

Philosophical & Ethical Justification for 15Minute.Fitness and Fit Families of Faith

I want to talk a little bit about the justification for our group, our program, and this book. Why Christian Moms and Dads—aren't all bodies the same? Of course. There is nothing unique about the biology of a Christian human body versus the human body of an atheist. But Christian parents are WHO we are, and therefore, they are our mission field.

"Mission Field" is the defining term, here. We see our coaching as a ministry—for health of the whole person—body and soul. My hero is St. Francis of Assisi. One of his quotes guides my life. He says, "Preach the Gospel at all times! And if necessary, use words."

The most powerful witness we will ever have is our lives—how we choose to live them. I want to model healthy behavior for those whom God has entrusted to my care. That is my cooperation with God's Providence. I want to help other Christian Moms and Dads model healthy behavior for their children.

If children saw more healthy role models, maybe then they might want to grow up to actually BE Christian Moms and Dads themselves. Instead, we see them more and more following the ways of modern society, which models broken families and faithlessness as the new "normal." We can fight this. We have to fight this. But, words are mere air tickling the ears. We must ACT. We must BE. We must model lives that our children respect and admire. This is how we "preach" most powerfully.

It could be argued that as Christians we are spiritual creatures, and therefore paying special attention to the body is ultimately counterproductive. I have heard this position. I understand it. And I am sympathetic to it. However, I do not share it. Here's why.

It is clear to me that the instant of my conception encompassed a two-fold gift—a brand new spirit was fused with a brand new body, neither of which had existed the moment before. Even taking into account the doctrine of original sin, it is certainly not the case that I was given a spirit by God and a body by Satan. No, God was the author of both, and what He gives is good.

It is not clear which one was given to me first. in fact, the most ancient Christian theological doctrine tells us that man is both spirit and flesh. True, St. Paul describes the internal moral conflict as a battle between the flesh and the spirit, but I think this points not toward some sort of fundamental evil nature of the body, but rather is an analogy to describe the seemingly impossible situation of being in conflict with oneself. After all, I am one single being. How can I be at odds with myself?

This is an ancient philosophical question (notably posed by Plato) which St. Paul picked up and examined theologically. I think using St. Paul's theological analogy as an excuse to ignore the health of the body is not defensible for the Christian. I am not a spirit who HAS a body. Neither am I a body which HAS a spirit. Rather, "I" am both, my body AND my spirit.

When I say "I" am hurt, I may be referring to either my spirit (emotional pain: sadness, heartbreak), or I may be referring to my body (physical pain: I stepped on a nail). Both my spirit and my body together make up WHAT I am as a human and WHO I am uniquely as an individual person. I do not exist and cannot function in the absence of either one of these two essential components of my being.

At the absolute least, I must admit that my body is my very first gift from God after I was brought into existence. If that is the case, do I not have a responsibility to care for, maintain, and provide for the flourishing of this primary gift from our heavenly father?

If your father gave you a new car, how do you think he would feel if you didn't take care of it? What if you neglected to change the oil or provide routine preventive maintenance? What if you fed it sewage instead of gasoline? What if you ignored it when the check engine light came on and continued to drive it without care, until it was rendered useless and was only worthy of the junkyard? Do you think your father would be very happy with you? Do you think this type of behavior shows respect and gratitude? Of course not.

I bet we can all agree that our bodies deserve at least as much care as our disposable vehicles. After all, we can't just go trade this body in on a new one at the year-end clearance sale. We're stuck with this one for the entirety of our life here on Earth. And when it ceases to work, we cease to live here.

With that in mind, I want to encourage you to begin this very day to look at your body in a new way. I hope you will look at it with gratitude. I hope you will look at it with a certain awe and holy fear. It is our very first gift from our Heavenly Father, and I want to help you make the most of your term of stewardship for this gift so that we may all here, "Well done good and faithful servant..."

And the best witness we can ever give to our children is to model healthy behavior. That includes spirit, mind AND body. God has shared his providential role in a special way with parents, who provide for the well-being of their children. Providing them with food, clothing and shelter takes care of their base survival needs right now, but that is a bare minimum. Forming their habits and their character is the highest level of service we can render them, molding them into good people who will live happy lives after they leave our homes and lead families of their own. Let's be the role models they deserve.

Our Heavenly Father didn't just tell us what to do, He showed us what to do when He took on human flesh and guided us personally. Let's imitate Him and do the same for our children. Let's SHOW them how to be whole, happy and healthy, so that they can show their children, and they can in turn show their children. We can be the turning point in the history of our entire lineage. Think about that. Let this realization sink in. Let this opportunity excite you. Let it motivate you to become the person you were meant to be, fully alive and in healthy balance of spirit, mind, and body.

Structure of this book

This book serves a couple of different purposes for a couple of different types of people in my community. First and foremost, it is a practical guide of action that allows you to follow simple steps week by week to move from point A to point B—from a point of ill-health to a point of good health and even athleticism, if you desire that.

Toward that end, the second section of this book is focused on action. If you simply desire to know the concrete step-by-step actions you need to take to follow this proven program in order to achieve new levels of health, fitness, strength, leanness and energy, then feel free to skip all the way to Part Two: "Action". It is a standalone guide to action that explains "WHAT to do and HOW to do it."

For those questioners out there (and I am very much one of you), the first section of this book is on theory. It gives the rationale, the arguments, and the conceptual basis for the action steps described in Part Two. It walks us through the "WHAT to do and WHY we should do it" questions.

I encourage you to follow the line of reasoning, to ask and attempt to answer the questions posed, and to judge for yourself whether or not you think this approach to permanent fat loss, health and fitness is the soundest, most practical and most reasonable path to take for you in your own personal circumstances of life. It is my belief that you will find ample justification to support the plan of action laid out in Section Two, and when you do move on to implement the theory from Section One, I hope you will refer back to this theoretical part to make sure you always have a good understanding of WHY you are doing what you're doing.

So, whether you are seeking theory, practice, or both, I hope you will find this book useful; and I hope you will use it as a tool for spiritual gratitude and self-development, for your own good, and for the good of those you love.

Resources to Help Along the Way

Many times in this book, you will find references to video instruction found within our Facebook™ community—Facebook Group "Fit Families of Faith" (facebook.com/groups/fitfamiliesoffaith), as well as our Facebook Business Page: "15 Minute Fitness" (facebook.com/15minutefit), and also our YouTube™ channel we are always updating: "15minute.fitness" (https://bit.ly/15minute_fitness_YouTube).

Links to all these can be found on our central hub, our website: www.15minute.fitness.

If you are not yet a member of our Facebook community, please do request to join. While the book is a standalone resource, sometimes there are concepts more easily demonstrable through video than through text-based communication alone. A picture is worth 1000 words, they say, and a video flashes 30 to 60 pictures a second, so imagine how many libraries worth of books it would take to house the information in a single video!

While that may be a bit of a stretch, the invitation and encouragement to join our group and watch the accompanying videos stands. I'm one for using all the tools in our toolbox that are helpful for getting the job done, and the instructional videos in are indeed useful tools toward that end.

While we're on the topic of tools, we at 15minute.fitness also advocate using a nutrition tracking app called Cronometer. There is a free version available for download on any smartphone platform. We like it better than MyFitnessPal, for instance, because it tracks not only calories and macro nutrients (protein, carbohydrates, and fat), but it also tracks micronutrients (vitamins and minerals). A hidden vitamin or mineral deficiency is pretty important information. It's necessary data in the picture of overall health. Thus, while you could track calories with MyFitnessPal, or even a pen and paper, Cronometer is hands-down a better tool for this job and the one for which we give explicit instructions inside our coaching program and inside this book.

I'm not telling you that you cannot gain muscle, lose weight, and improve your health without using Cronometer. But I am telling you that it is a really useful tool for this job. Certainly, you could build a house without using a hammer, a saw, or power tools; but you can build a better house, faster if you do use the best tools available for the job at hand. So, as we give instructions in this book, I will lay them out with reference to using power tools, i.e. Cronometer. You are totally free not to use it, but you will have to tailor my instructions to your tool of choice.

PART I

THERORETICAL FOUNDATIONS

CHAPTER 1
THE PROBLEM

Self-diagnosis

nosce te ipsum (know thyself)

This section is on self-diagnosis. It is important to know exactly where you are in terms of beginning point before you are able to plot a course to your intended destination. So, I want you to imagine a line with five dots on it.

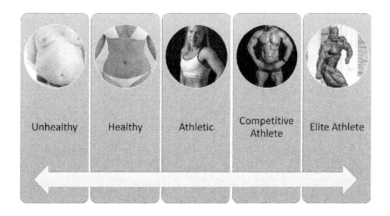

This represents the fitness continuum. The left side of the line begins with a dot labeled "Unhealthy". This represents a condition of being far from your ideal body weight and at risk for obesity-related illnesses, like diabetes, hypertension, heart attack and stroke. The next dot to the right represents "Healthy". Healthy is the condition in which you are close to your ideal body weight and not at risk for obesity-related illnesses. The third dot his "Athletic". This is a level of physical conditioning proper to athletes. Here, you have achieved muscular definition and leanness through regular exercise, and people can tell that you work out by your appearance. The fourth dot to the right is labeled "Competitive Athlete". This represents a level of physical conditioning appropriate to an athlete to be competitive in physique competitions. You are able to compete regularly, effectively and competently. And the last dot at the end of the line is "Elite athlete". This simply means that you compete at the top 10% of physique competitions.

It is vitally important that you find yourself somewhere

in this continuum. Then, you need to know your end goal. The only way you can effectively plot a course from point A to point B is to know where your starting point is and where your end goal is. Otherwise, how can you possibly hope to get there? The only place you will get, without first finding your bearings, is lost.

It's crucial to this process that you find yourself on this continuum, that you find your starting point. It takes very different tools, tactics and techniques to move from one point of the continuum to another at the various levels. For instance, it takes a different set of dietary practices and training protocols to move from the level of "competitive athlete" to "elite level athlete" than it does to move from the level of "unhealthy" to "healthy". And different coaches specialize in addressing different parts of this continuum.

My coaching program, and this book, specializes in moving people from a state of "unhealthy" to "healthy" or "athletic". I'm not terribly interested in helping a competitive athlete put an extra half inch on their biceps, an extra two inches on their vertical jump, shave two-tenths of a second off their 40 yard dash, or put another 10 pounds on their bench press. There is nothing wrong with those goals, and every competitive athlete wants to improve, but that's not where my heart is. My passion lies in helping normal Christian families have healthier, happier lives.

If you are a competitive athlete trying to reach elite level status, I will happily refer you to coaches who specialize in particular sports skills and competition prep. If you are at the level of unhealthy and you would like to move to the level of healthy, or beyond that to athletic, then I am the coach for you. This book will outline the most effective and time-efficient approach to attaining those goals, while living real lives with real families and real responsibilities.

Personally, just as a point of reference for this continuum, I would consider myself at the level of "competitive athlete". I could walk on stage for a physique competition and feel at home there. I might not win or even crack the top five, depending on the field of competitors, but neither would I be dead last. Having myself moved from the level of "unhealthy" to "healthy" and "athletic" to "competitive athlete", I am very happy in my own skin. And having coached many others successfully along the same path, I have found my mode of serving God and loving my neighbor here on this earth. For the opportunity to help you, the reader, along this journey, I am truly and eternally grateful.

How do I see my role as coach in the overall landscape of healthy, fit and happy lives? I see my role as different from, but in tandem with, medical doctors. However, I think the present environment in western medicine has put the cart before the horse. Here's what I mean:

Common practice in western medicine today is to assess the patient at the symptomatic level. Procedures or pharmaceuticals are prescribed to alleviate the symptoms of diseased conditions. The underlying disorder is acknowledged, but it is met at, and restricted to, the level of symptoms—effects rather than causes.

I see my job as coach to move people from an overall state of unhealthy to healthy. I teach and guide people toward their ideal body weight and a healthy body fat percentage. This, in turn, restores order to the body. It does away with the many causes of the diseases which produced the symptoms in the first place—the symptoms that western medicine tends to focus on and address.

I see my role as presenting an intervention which addresses the causes rather than the effects. The body has an amazing ability to heal itself when everything is working in the proper order, when it is in a state of health. If, after achieving a state of health, symptoms persist, then doctors should be employed to look for more obscure causes of those symptoms. By that point, lifestyle factors and obesity will have been ruled out.

It is my thesis that the very first intervention in terms of helping individuals should be a systematic program which moves them from a state of unhealthy to healthy. At that point, the medical community can more easily discern the types of problems fixable by their field, rather than being confused and confounded by the simple state of being in a general, overall state of ill-health.

Can you imagine how much less money would be spent on health care in this country if the first intervention were not to impose a life sentence of pharmaceuticals on an obviously obese individual? Can you imagine how many lives would be saved by prescribing a treatment that actually addresses the underlying problem? Can you imagine how many lives would be improved if there were real help out there to provide structured and simple steps to move someone from a point of unhealthy to healthy? This is the gap I'm seeking to fill.

Interventions

This program assumes that you are not currently at the peak of health. If, right now, you are in the absolute best shape of your life and you are making continual progress, I don't want to get in the way of whatever is working for you. I am very much of the opinion that if something is not broke, it doesn't need fixing. The last thing I want to do is to confuse someone who is already on the right track. If that is you, then put this book away somewhere safely and only access it if you find yourself stuck and needing to get moving in the right direction again.

Most of you reading this book have already come to the conclusion that your level of health and fitness is not exactly where you would like it to be. If that is you, then please read this book all the way through, as it will present the most effective intervention possible. This intervention will change your life forever. It is not a short-term diet that will cause you to drop a bunch of water weight in a week's time (which comes right back), and it is not a short-term exercise plan that you can't keep up for the long haul. Rather, the intervention I am presenting here is the best possible investment of your time and energy, returning to you the absolute most benefits in terms of the efforts asked from you. Within these pages is the overall lifestyle plan for permanent bodily health and complete transformation.

So, what is the thrust of this message? Well, you can already intuit that any state of ill-health requires some sort of intervention. If you've noticed, I've used the term intervention many times in the last few paragraphs. Why? An intervention is a short-term prescription to alleviate a particular problem, while an overall lifestyle plan is something you carry on long-term. Which one am I advocating? Both.

This program constitutes an overall lifestyle plan which is made up of specific interventions to address specific problems that arise in terms of health and fitness. The primary audience for this book largely finds themselves in an overfat condition. So, the question is what sort of intervention is optimum to alleviate this?

Any intervention, if it is to be successful, must address the one underlying universal condition by which fat is burned off the body, energy balance.

Energy Balance Equation:

(A Calorie is simply a unit of measure for energy—just like an inch is a unit of measure for length)

Calories-in = Calories-out
(Eucaloric or Maintenance Diet—energy taken in just meets the needs of the body.)

Calories-in > Calories-out
(Hypercaloric Diet—energy taken in exceeds the body's needs; the extra will likely be stored as body fat.)

Calories-in < Calories-out
(Hypocaloric Diet—energy taken in is inadequate for body's needs; energy will have to be taken from stored body fat.)

Energy balance is a fancy way of describing the equation of calories-in versus calories-out. When the two sides of that equation are balanced, you take in as many calories as you expend. No extra energy is stored as body fat, and you achieve homeostasis. Your body is in a state of maintenance and it remains as it is. When you take in more calories than you expend, your body stores that extra energy somewhere. The form of storage which concerns us here is storage of energy in the form of visceral or body fat. I could dedicate a chapter to all of the ill health effects and disease risks associated with increased levels of visceral and body fat, but I don't think you would have read this far if you didn't already recognize that as a problem for which you are seeking a solution.

Any sort of effective intervention which seeks to tap into stores of visceral and body fat must manipulate that energy balance equation in the other direction. We must attempt to expend more calories than we take in. It's really like your household budget. If you don't bring in enough dollars to pay the bills, then you have to tap into your savings account in order to make up the difference. It is the same with energy. If you don't bring in enough calories through your diet to fuel your body's needs, then your body must access the stored energy in your fat reserves to make up for the shortfall. And, if we are over fat, that is exactly what we want to do.

So, the question is: what is the best way to shift that energy balance equation into our favor? Well, there are only two sides of the equation, so there are only two variables to manipulate: calories-in and calories-out. We can restrict the calories-in side by eating a low-calorie diet. And we can increase the calories-out side by using strategies to make our bodies burn more calories.

CHAPTER 2
FAILED ATTEMPTS

Diet & Cardio

Now, let's have a look at two of the most common interventions employed toward this end: Diet and Cardiovascular Exercise. Let's take a closer look and how each of these tools addresses the energy balance equation.

A low-calorie diet reduces the calories-in side of the equation, and for it to be effective, it must reduce it below the level of the calories-out side. A low-calorie diet will normally be the backbone of any effective fat loss intervention. That's because it is much easier to meaningfully reduce the calories you take into your body than to meaningfully raise the amount of calories you burn. For instance, a peanut butter and jelly sandwich has over 400 calories. For a normal sized person, it would take about two hours on the treadmill to burn that many calories. Which is more feasible: To forgo a peanut butter sandwich or to dedicate 2 hours to a treadmill every day? The effect on the energy balance equation is the same.

The relative ease with which we can change the balance of the equation through restricting calories in our diet versus trying to change the balance of the equation by increasing energy expenditure through activity is why the low-calorie diet holds first place in terms of losing fat.

However, it is not without its own set of problems. The primary problem is that it is relatively short-lived. The longer we remain in a caloric deficit, the more our bodies adapt to functioning in a lower-calorie environment, and our metabolisms slow down. If you have ever done a low-calorie diet for an extended period of time, I have no doubt that you have experienced this. Sooner or later your body stopped losing fat. No matter how few calories you ate, your body simply refused to give up any more visceral or body fat. Our body is remarkably adaptive and suited for survival. It has built-in defense mechanisms against death by starvation, aimed at reducing caloric needs in times of caloric deprivation. Thus, there is a time-limit built into the effectiveness of a low-calorie diet for fat loss.

So, what about the other popular approach? What about increasing energy expenditure through cardio?

As previously stated, there are two sides to the energy balance equation, and you can certainly manipulate the calories-out side by increasing energy expenditure through activity. Even if we keep our caloric intake the same, we can theoretically raise the energy-out side enough to shift the balance of the equation towards fat loss.

Cardio is often used toward this end for a couple of reasons. It requires virtually no extra equipment. One can simply go outside and take a walk. Also, it is a low-intensity activity that can be kept up for a relatively long time. You can burn a fairly significant amount of calories while barely breaking a sweat or getting out of breath, if you extend the duration of your activity over a couple of hours. It doesn't take an intense level of effort. It extends the effort over a prolonged period of time. It takes a great deal of time, but not a great deal of effort.

However, as mentioned above, the actual amount of calories that you can expend through exercise alone is pretty small. In the example from the section on low calorie diets, two hours on a treadmill is equal to a single peanut butter sandwich. In order to lose a pound of body fat each week using cardio alone to manipulate the energy balance equation would require Over 17 hours on that treadmill each week. That's a lot of time.

Why Do We Regain Weight?

Now, let's look at the end result. We'll assume a successful intervention in terms of fat loss for each of the above approaches, a low-calorie diet or cardio.

First, let's assume you restricted your calories through diet over several months and lost 15 pounds of body fat. As we discussed, your body has adapted to the low-calorie state and reached homeostasis. Your metabolism has slowed to a crawl, and you have ceased losing fat. What happens next? If you continue the low-calorie diet, your metabolism will continue to grind down to a death-crawl, and your hormone levels will crash. This is due to the well-documented phenomenon called "metabolic adaptation", universally acknowledged in the scientific literature. Restrict your body's energy intake for prolonged periods and it will adapt, looking for every way possible to conserve energy, to stretch every calorie to the maximum possible extent, to adapt itself to a low-calorie condition...ultimately, to not-die.

Your body will literally be in starvation mode, you will feel like you have no energy, and your body will be craving nutrition from which it has been deprived for the last several months. Not only is this an unhealthy state to be in, but it is a perfect setup for regaining the weight you lost.

In order to heal your metabolism, rebalance your hormones and restore some semblance of health, you will need to eat. And when you begin eating again, what should we expect to happen? Your body has adapted to maintaining its weight on a very low-calorie intake, let's say a thousand calories a day for the sake of illustration. If 1000 calories a day is your new maintenance level (where calories-in = calories-out), what happens when you begin eating 1500 calories a day? Well, at least initially, until your body begins healing and adapting, you will store those extra 500 calories a day in your storage tank: visceral and body fat. There you go regaining the fat you suffered so long to lose.

Now let's assume you had a successful intervention for fat loss by increasing your caloric expenditure through cardio. You dedicated those 17 hours a week on a treadmill, and over the course of 20 weeks, you lost 20 pounds of fat. We won't even mention the fact that as your cardiovascular health improved you actually become more efficient in converting calories into activity and therefore get diminishing returns in terms of calorie burning from the same level of activity. (You got BETTER at squeezing energy from every calorie you take in, driving your maintenance calorie level even lower.) Rather, we will ask the more practical question: can you reliably and consistently dedicate 17 hours a week on a treadmill for the rest of your life?

If cardio was your intervention, the mechanism you used in order to shift the energy balance equation in your favor and lose those 20 pounds, then your answer better be "yes" if you want to keep the weight off. What happens when you cease to give those two hours a day to increasing your energy expenditure? Well, the calories-out side of the equation then falls short of the calories-in, and we know that it is by definition the formula for storing those extra calories as visceral and body fat. If you lost fat through a cardio intervention, then you better be able to keep up that cardio intervention for life if you want to maintain your weight loss. Congratulations, you have become a slave to your treadmill!

By now, you can start to see why so many interventions fail over the long term. Even if they are successful during the actual intervention, there is no compelling reason for your body not to go back to its previous state after the intervention is over. You have done nothing to fundamentally change your metabolism. You manipulated the energy balance equation for a short time, but you did nothing to alter either the calories-in side or the calories-out side of the equation going forward.

I want to introduce you to a better way...

CHAPTER 3
THE SOLUTION

Muscle-Building

There is indeed a better way, an approach that is more effective in the short term and more sustainable over time. First, let's step back and examine the energy (or calorie) needs of our bodies.

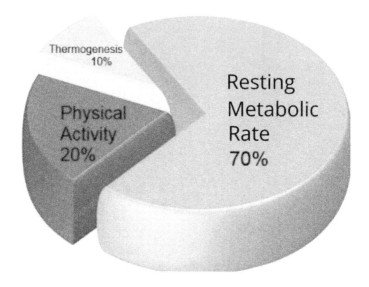

In the pie chart above, the largest portion denotes the percentage of your daily caloric expenditure for your Resting Metabolic Rate (RMR). This is the amount of calories your body expends at rest, simply idling. The mid-sized portion represents the amount of calories that we expend through physical activity, and the smallest portion is the amount of calories used, and dissipated as heat, through digesting food.

As you can see, the vast majority of the calories you expend each day is from your Resting Metabolic Rate (RMR). The first two interventions we discussed, low-calorie diets and cardio, focus on the smallest proportions of your daily caloric expenditure. While they can work, they do nothing (or even negatively impact) the largest driver of total daily calorie burn, the resting metabolic rate. And after those types of intervention are over, your resting metabolic rate is either unchanged or actually suppressed.

What if there were a way to increase your largest driver of total daily caloric expenditure—your Resting Metabolic Rate? What if instead of suppressing my biggest calorie burner, I could actually ramp it up and increase the rate at which I burn calories on a daily basis while simply existing? And because the resting metabolic rate is, by definition, the amount of calories I burn at rest; what if I could increase that amount by a significant margin, the number of calories I burn while sitting on the couch or sleeping? Wouldn't that be amazing? But that sounds too good to be true—pure fantasy, right? Wrong.

It's actually relatively simple. Build muscle.

How does building muscle change things? Muscle burns calories at rest. Muscle does not only burn calories during intentional physical activity, like cardio. No, muscle burns calories merely by existing. The more muscle you have, the more calories you burn while doing nothing.

Think about it like this. Your body is like a mechanical system, like a car. What does body fat do? Nothing. It basically has no activity. Your body fat reserves are simply storage places for extra energy, like the carrying gas cans in the trunk of your car. The body fat you carry is analogous to junk in your trunk. it just sits there. You can open up the trunk and get some out when you need it, but it doesn't do anything while sitting in storage.

Now, muscle is very active. Anything your body does is as a result of some muscle or other contracting and relaxing. It's like the motor of your car. It's the thing responsible for all activity. And it even burns gas (calories) at idle. If you don't believe this, go crank up your car and leave it idling in your driveway overnight. See if it still has gas in the tank when you wake up tomorrow morning. Just like the motor in your car, muscle burns calories at idle. You don't have to intentionally do anything, it just constantly uses energy. And the bigger your motor, the more gas it uses.

So, to extend this analogy, how does cardio attempt to burn more calories? Basically, cardio is like driving for a long time with a four-cylinder engine. With a small four-cylinder, you need to drive a long way for a long time to burn a gallon of gas.

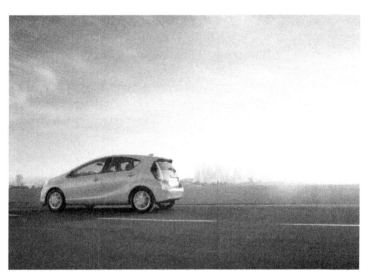

In contrast, an eight-cylinder engine will burn the same amount of gas on a much shorter drive. And if you leave them both running in your driveway side by side, which one do you think will burn through a gallon of gas quicker while idling?

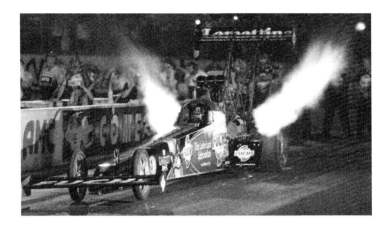

The bigger engine burns more gas all the time, active or idling. The bigger muscle will burn more calories whether engaged in voluntary activity or merely at rest, idling on the sofa.

This is the secret to effective, long-term body change. Building a bigger motor causes you to burn more gas forever, even at rest. As long as you have a big engine in your car, it is going to be a gas hog. The same is true with muscle. Building more muscle causes you to burn more calories at rest forever. In terms of the pie-chart we looked at, you will effectively raise your resting metabolic rate, the single biggest factor in the amount of calories you burn every single day. And that equates to more gas burned, more calories expended, day in and day out, week in and week out, without any special extra activity—forever. You simply have to build, and maintain, an increased amount of skeletal muscle tissue. That's it.

Cardio doesn't do that, and neither does a low-calorie restricted diet. That's why those sorts of interventions only work in the short-term. They don't build you a bigger motor, so when you try to eat some of the things that normal people eat, you get fat again. Or, when you try to reclaim some of your daily time, when you can't devote two hours a day to a treadmill anymore, you get fat again. You haven't built a bigger motor. You haven't changed your resting metabolic rate. So, you should expect to put the fat back on when the intervention is over. Why wouldn't you?

Now that we've examined the components of our daily caloric expenditure, identified the biggest and most important piece, resting metabolic rate, and identified how to increase that factor by building muscle, all we have to figure out now is how to go about it.

But wait, cardio can still affect energy-out through activity. Shouldn't I do that too?

I get asked this all the time by well-meaning (but impatient) clients who are rightfully enthusiastic about getting in shape. After all, even if it is ONLY 20% of your daily caloric expenditure, that's not insignificant. Calories-out through activity still works, right?

Yes, but...even here, merely in terms of calories burned DURING the workout, resistance training just destroys cardio as a calorie-burning activity in itself.

Burning Calories inside the workout (comparison):

Resistance training burns far more calories per unit of time than does cardio. The reason is that they use two different energy pathways. Cardio exercise utilizes aerobic respiration to turn the energy we eat (calories) into energy we can use (ATP). Resistance training of the type advocated here in our program utilizes the glycolytic energy pathway to make the same conversion (calories$\rightarrow$ ATP).

The main difference between these two pathways for us is the relative efficiencies. Aerobic respiration is far more efficient in this conversion than is glycolysis—about 15 times more efficient. That means that for every unit of energy-in (calories), aerobic respiration produces 15 times more units of ATP than does glycolysis.

But efficiency is good, right? Well...let's think about what we are trying to do. We are trying to unbalance the energy balance equation—tilt it in the direction of fewer calories-in and more calories-out. We are trying to use as many calories as possible—not conserve them and spend them very efficiently and miserly.

It is as if our goal is to SPEND money—as much money as possible so that we have to dip into our savings account (our fat reserves) to supply the difference. If that is the case, I want to be inefficient; I want to be a spendthrift! I want to overpay for everything. For aerobic respiration (very efficient), I can buy 15 units of usable energy for the low price of one dollar! With glycolysis, those same 15 units of energy cost me $15! That would be terrible if I was trying to save money, but it is wonderful if I am trying to spend calories!

That's super-efficient, and it would probably save my life if I was dying of starvation—trying to squeeze the absolute most out of every precious calorie I could scrape from beneath the nearest rock. But, I'm an overfed, modern American. I have the exact opposite problem! I have easy access to far more calories than I actually need for activity. Obesity-related diseases are killing far more people in western society today than starvation.

If I rely on aerobic respiration to be my mechanism to increase calories-out, I have to burn 15 times the amount of ATP to consume the same number of calories. That's a lot of treadmill time! And while treadmill time is relatively easy compared to lifting heavy objects, I prefer to give a bit more effort in order to save a lot more time! I'm just not going to spend 15 minutes on a treadmill to burn the same amount of calories I could have burned in one minute lifting weights. My time is too precious.

Post-workout

So, resistance training uses far more calories per unit of time during the workout than cardio, but what about after the workout? Again, let's do what we always do...let's examine it!

After a cardio workout, what state is your body in? Well, you're tired. But, as soon as your heart rate returns to normal, your metabolism also returns to normal. It doesn't have anything new or extra to do. After your heart stops beating fast, you are in the same state as you were before you spent your hours on the treadmill.

After an intelligently designed resistance-training workout, you have activated muscle protein synthesis. What is that? It is a technical term denoting the bodily process of converting dietary protein into muscle tissue. It is the muscle-building process.

You see, you do not add muscle tissue in the gym while working out. In the gym, you only flip a switch and activate a process (muscle protein synthesis). This bodily process goes on for the next 24-48 hours while you rest. As a process, it costs energy—it takes calories to fuel this process. It also takes raw materials (amino acids in protein) to form new muscle tissue. Where do these come from? They come from the protein you eat.

So, you've burned more calories per unit of time while in the gym, you've initiated a bodily process which goes on for the next 24 – 48 hours, and this process requires extra protein from the food you eat as well as extra miscellaneous calories to be converted into ATP to fuel this process. And the end result of this process is more muscle tissue on your frame which then raises your resting metabolic rate—the biggest piece of the daily caloric expenditure pie chart (by far).

Do you see an entire chain of events that come together to tilt the energy balance equation in your favor? It really is the perfect storm we have all been searching for to move our bodies from overfat to lean for life!

It really is the difference between spending your time and investing your time. You can spend your time on a treadmill, get an immediate reward (calories burned) and have no lasting effect. You only get a similar benefit tomorrow if you spend your time over again.

Or, you can invest your time resistance training, which also gives an immediate reward (calories burned), but continues to give for the next 24 – 48 hours (MPS), plus pays dividends for the rest of your life (raises your RMR). I don't know about you, but this seems like a no-brainer to me.

How?

Ultimately, it is the actual mass of muscle tissue which most closely correlates with increasing resting metabolic rate. In other words, what we are trying to achieve is increasing muscle size rather than focusing on endurance or strength. While there is a good deal of overlap between those goals, keeping our eyes fixed on the specific goal of increasing muscle size will help us choose the most important and most effective techniques and strategies, without getting sidetracked on things of lesser importance.

For instance, cross training, training for several different goals at once, will not be as effective for body composition change as a laser-focused effort on one specific goal at a time. And the first specific goal you should aim for if you want to achieve lower body fat levels forever is building bigger muscles, adding skeletal muscle tissue to your frame. Thus, we will include the steps necessary to achieve that goal and exclude anything which diverts our focus for the time being.

This doesn't mean we will never focus on pure strength or pure endurance. It just means that we will only do so after the present, most important intervention. First of all, we must fix our problem with body fat. Let's focus on the most important thing first, and see what other aspects of our life are changed as a result. Endurance, health and strength will all progress as a side effect, and then we can more sharply focus on other things we want to improve.

Usually, getting the body into a healthy body fat percentage range fixes the vast majority of health problems and health markers that act as predictors for future disease. Getting the body into a healthy body fat percentage range increases our strength and endurance, enhances our energy level, appearance and self-confidence, and pretty much covers all of our bases.

So, what methodology do we use to build bigger muscles?

If you grew up in my generation, and if you were a fan of bodybuilding, you probably listened to people like Arnold Schwarzenegger, who was famous for saying "No pain, no gain!" and "You have to break down the muscle in order to build it back up."

Well, now we are blessed to live in an age where sport

and exercise science is constantly examining and studying all aspects of human performance and improvement on a vast scale. The things Arnold Schwarzenegger did worked for him because he was a genetic anomaly and because he and others had stumbled upon a few of the basic principles that build muscle, even while applying them unsystematically by trial and error.

What sport Science has done over the last decade is precisely to uncover the root causes that actually serve to build muscle and to attempt to codify and give some sort of systematic guidance in the application of those fundamental principles. In our coaching programs, we bring these discoveries and guidelines down from the level of scientific research and elite athletics, and make them fit into the lives of real people—specifically busy Christian moms and dads who want to improve their health and fitness and who want to model healthy behavior for their children, and their children's children... These are the people for whom this book is written. If that is you, read on.

aMPS™

The physiological process of muscle-building at the cellular level is called muscle protein synthesis, MPS. Muscle is made of protein, so muscle protein synthesis is simply a fancy term to denote the process of turning dietary protein, the protein you eat in food, into skeletal muscle tissue on your body. So, what we need to do is to trigger muscle protein synthesis in order to put our body into a muscle-building state.

That's where aMPS come in. "aMPS" is our super-cool word for a Muscle Protein Synthesis activator. We activate muscle protein synthesis in 15-minute workouts called aMPS.

We now know that you do not need to break down the muscle in order to build it back up. Exercise science tells us that's not how it works. In fact, "breaking down" muscle tissue is the last thing we want to do. Muscle damage requires all of our recuperative ability simply to heal back up to the original condition. That's like digging a hole in order to build up a hill— counterproductive. That's working backwards, working against yourself.

Thus, there is no need to brutalize your body with hours of training with heavy weights. Rather, you simply need to provide enough mechanical tension on a particular muscle group to trigger muscle protein synthesis. An intelligently designed workout can get this done in 15 minutes. And an intelligently designed workout regimen can provide this stimulus for all the major muscle groups in your body with several 15-minute amps spread out over the course of a week. That's what we do.

"aMPS" trigger muscle protein synthesis which will last anywhere from 24 to 48 hours. To ensure that the body is continually in a muscle-building state as opposed to a fat-storing state, we advise using aMPS every 24-48 hours. In practical terms, this means we advise doing a 15-minute aMPS workout every day if possible.

Think about it this way, 15 minutes is technically 1% of your day. Can you devote 1% of your day to the health and fitness of your body? If not, can you really say your health is a priority in your life?

In full disclosure, Jackie and I always schedule Sundays as off days. We have church and Sunday lunch with the extended family. It's a day of rest and relaxation, communion with God and with family. So, we never work out on Sundays. Because we split all the major muscle groups into three different workouts which we call "Push workout", "Pull workout", and "Legs workout", six days on and one day off works out perfectly. We stimulate each major muscle group twice over a week's time and take a full rest day. It fits our lives, and it works. We help our clients find ways to make it fit their lives, and it definitely works for them. It can fit your life and work for you too.

Workout Regimen Structure

There are literally thousands of exercises out there and almost as many ways to group them. I'll move on to exercise selection in a moment, but first let's discuss how we should organize particular workouts into a comprehensive regimen.

Let me begin with the general and then drill down into particulars. In general, there are two types of resistance training regimens: 1) a "full-body" routine, which presents a challenge to all your muscle groups in a single workout session; and 2) a "split" routine, which splits all your muscle groups into two or more separate exercise sessions.

Advantages of a full body routine are as follows:

1.   You can work every muscle group in a single gym session.
2.   You could potentially stimulate each muscle group more times per week for the same total number of workout sessions.
3.   Requires lower frequency—one single workout can cover all your muscle groups.

Disadvantages to full body routines:

1.   They make for long workouts (it takes longer to work every muscle group in a session than to only work a portion of your muscle groups).
2.   You cannot keep up optimal intensity for long periods, so exercises placed later in that session are not as effective as exercises done earlier in the session when you were "fresh" and full of energy. We get worn out.
3.   Because the quality of your effort diminishes over the lengthy exercise session, the later sets are

called by exercise scientists "junk volume"—sets that aren't above the level-of-effort threshold necessary to stimulate muscle protein synthesis. (Spinning your wheels, these waste your time with "busy work" for no physiological purpose related to our goals).

4.   It easily leads to overtraining and central nervous system (CNS) fatigue—especially as we get older, and our recuperative abilities wane.

5.   Long exercise sessions sap your energy (you've given your all in the gym—there's nothing left for real life outside the gym).

Advantages of a split routine:

1.   Workouts can be much shorter in duration (it does not take as long to challenge a subset of all muscle groups).

2.   You can bring full intensity to every rep of every set of every exercise before you tire out.

3.   Thus, every rep of every set "counts"—they are effective. No wasted effort. No wasted time. Efficiency.

4.   Gives particular muscle groups a chance to rest and recover while continuing to stimulate other muscle groups, keeping your body in a constant state of muscle protein synthesis rather than being in fat-storage mode.

Disadvantages:

1.   Requires higher frequency—it takes multiple exercise sessions to cover all the major muscle groups.

Discussion:

Both can be viable models, and I have used (and do use both on occasion). I did a week of full-body workouts recently when I began exercising again after having

Covid. There is a time and place for each of the tools in our toolbox, and both these models are merely tools for the end of presenting challenges to muscle groups in order to grow muscle.

That said, I rarely program full-body workouts (except for absolute beginners or briefly after a long layoff), and I think for 90% of people 90% of the time, a split routine is superior.

Physiology is the major factor. By splitting my muscle groups into parts, I can work SOMETHING every day. Properly challenging a muscle triggers muscle protein synthesis (MPS), which lasts anywhere from 24-48 hours. By working out every day (or maybe even every other day), I can stay continually in MPS. Thus, my body is perpetually in a muscle-building state. This (constant MPS) effectively grows muscle faster, uses more energy (muscle-building is a metabolically "expensive" activity; it uses a lot of calories), and keeps me out of a fat-storing mode.

Time is also a factor. It is easier for me to find 15 minutes sometime during the day than to dedicate an hour or more to a workout. And as half that hour-long workout is wasted effort (see disadvantages to full-body sessions above), I just don't have room for that kind of wasted time and energy in my life.

Energy is a factor. I want to get energy OUT of my workout—not devote all my energy TO my workout. A long workout leaves me tired. A short workout energizes me and gets me pumped for the rest of my day—for "real" life outside the gym.

Ultimately, we must view these as tools. There are different tools for different goals and different sets of parameters. When you have a fully-stocked toolbox, you can pull out the proper tool for the proper task at the proper time. I am not against full-body routines. I use them myself occasionally. The real goal is to stock your toolbox with tools and then gain knowledge and experience on how and when to use each one.

That said, I think the vast majority of people will benefit more from more frequent 15 minute workouts than fewer, less effective hour-long sessions. Thus, my recommendation and instructions in this book will advocate a split routine.

The most common split routines are "Upper/Lower", which split your muscle groups into two categories—upper body and lower body; "Push/Pull/Legs", which further split your upper body muscle groups according to function—"pushing" away from your body and "pulling" towards your body. And "Bro-Splits" (a term referring to the normal gym "bro" in your local gym), which divide the muscle groups individually (e.g. Arm Day, Shoulder Day, Chest Day, Back Day, Leg Day...).

Bro-splits are generally looked down upon by exercise scientists and evidence-based practitioners as overly specialized and without backing by research. You just don't need an entire exercise session devoted to a single muscle group. Upper/Lower and Push/Pull/Legs have firmer bases in the research. I organize my routines along both lines, though I tend to favor Push/Pull/Legs most of the time. It fits very nicely with our present schema, so this is the split I will discuss and set up here in this book. So, we'll devise three workouts: 1) Push, 2) Pull and 3) Legs.

I will begin each of these sections on particular workouts with a general discussion on mechanics. It is important for you to understand the basic mechanical patterns for each movement so that you can select particular exercises that fit. I don't know what equipment you have available, so I will describe the movement pattern we are desiring inside these workouts and then give some example exercises which all fit that pattern. Don't overcomplicate it. Lifting body weight, dumbbells, barbells, rocks, bags of books, buckets of water, gallons of milk, resistance bands—all can provide mechanical tension on the muscle. And, the particular exercise you select is of only marginal importance. They are mostly interchangeable as long as you follow the movement pattern and present a real challenge (in terms of level of effort) to the targeted muscle groups.

1.   "Push" Workout: This describes movements of the upper body which push away from you. There are basically two planes of motion to cover: a horizontal push (pushing straight out from your chest) and a vertical push (pushing something up over your head). These are the two movement patterns we need to cover in the Push workout. Choose one exercise for each movement pattern.

Exercise selection examples:
(Horizontal Push) Bench Press, Pushup
(Vertical Press) Dumbbell Overhead Press

Major muscle groups worked include the chest (pectoralis), shoulders (anterior and medial deltoids) and arms (triceps).

2.   "Pull" Workout: This describes movements of the upper body which pull towards you. Again, there are basically two planes of movement to cover: a horizontal pull (pulling in toward your chest) and a

vertical pull (pulling upward from waste level to shoulder level). [If you have the capability to incorporate a downward pull—such as pull-down or chinup—there might be some merit to add that, or rotate it out with the horizontal pull. If you don't have access to equipment for that—a cable tower or pullup bar, don't worry about it.]

Exercise selection examples:
(Horizontal Pull) Bent over Row, Band Row, [Pullups]
(Vertical Pull) Upright Row

Major muscle groups worked include the back (latissimus dorsi, trapezius, spinal erectors), shoulders (posterior and medial deltoids) and arms (biceps).

3. "Leg" Workout: This will encompass movements of the lower body. Again, there are basically types of movement to cover: a squatting movement (think pushing away from your body with your legs) and a hip-hinge movement ("pulling" your hips into line with your torso). [Some leg exercises (like lunges) really fall into both categories, so they may be used for either].

Exercise selection examples:
(Squatting Movement) Squats, Leg Press, Lunges
(Hip-Hinge Movement) Stiff-legged Deadlift, Glute Bridge, Lunges

Major muscle groups worked include the legs (quadriceps and hamstrings) and the butt (gluteus medius and maximus).

[I don't program direct ab work as they are engaged strongly in most all movements when you really challenge yourself with the resistance. Few people really need to grow their waistline, anyway. Usually, we just need to reduce the fat there if we want to see a six-pack or a flat tummy. Abs really are "made in the kitchen." You'll also see there is no direct calf work here. If we walk a little more than usual, this is usually sufficient stimulus for calf development.]

Progression

In order to continually stimulate your muscles to adapt and grow, you have to continually provide a greater challenge to those muscles. some sort of progression over the course of time is necessary to stimulate further adaptations. For instance, let's say I do 10 push-ups today. Let's say that was enough to challenge my muscles to grow and force them to adapt. I might only be able to do 10 push-ups again on my next workout, perhaps even on the one after that. But sooner or later, my muscles will grow and adapt to the stimulus provided by 10 push-ups. Then, they require a stronger stimulus.

If I am still only doing ten pushups a year from now, then you can be sure that my body will look the same then as it does now. Why wouldn't it? If you have ever had a gym membership for any length of time, you have probably seen the same people lifting the same weights year after year. There is no wonder they look the same year after year. They have not done anything to force their bodies to change. They have achieved homeostasis.

When your muscles adapt to a certain level of stimulus, then that level of stimulus no longer forces your muscles to change. They already changed. They already adapted. They are now suited to handle to those ten push-ups. if I want them to keep changing, I have to provide progressively more challenge. I have to progress the amount of mechanical tension I apply to those muscles.

Progression can take many forms. However, the main variables are sets, reps and weight used. You can do more reps with the same weight for the same number of sets. Or you can hold reps constant and add weight for the same number of sets. Or you can hold reps constant and weight constant and add more sets. Those are the three main variables in play in terms of resistance training. Increasing any one of those provides more stimulus for muscle protein synthesis over time. So, you must make sure that the overall course of our workout regimen includes some sort of progression over time if you want to continually lead your body to further change.

We do this in our program in several steps. The first step is always a focus on exercise frequency. I want our clients to incorporate aMPS into their daily life. This gets a 15-minute workout stimulating muscle protein synthesis every single day.

Usually, step number two will address level of effort (intensity). There's a certain threshold in terms of level of effort below which muscle simply is not built. Think about cardio for instance. Have you ever seen a marathon runner with big muscles? No, they are normally extremely skinny. That's because jogging does not provide an intense enough stimulus for muscles to grow in size. it is a low-intensity activity which can be carried on for hours at a time. 15 minutes of jogging-level intensity will not reach the minimum threshold to build muscle.

So, after we get exercise frequency built into people's lives, I then asked them to increase their level of effort. Even though we're only exercising 15 minutes, it should be a difficult and challenging 15 minutes. Every rep of every set is important, and at the second stage of the exercise regimen, I asked people to pay attention to their last five reps of every set. These last five reps should be difficult, and you should never stop an exercise if you think you could have done several more reps. At stage two of the program, I ask clients to balance reps and weight to a level where they can fully tire themselves out on each set. That's the second way I build progression into a client program: intensity.

Once people have found a challenging weight to use for a suitable number of reps in each set, how then do we proceed? If our focus was pure strength, we would then continue adding weight every single workout every single week. Why? That is the definition of strength, moving the maximum amount of weight possible. But that's not our immediate goal, remember? We want to focus on muscle size. And believe it or not, training for size is slightly different than training for pure strength.

So, once I have coached clients to give a suitable level of effort to every single workout, the next way I like to progress their routine is by adding sets. This increases the total volume of work they do, a technical term in exercise science denoting Sets x Weight x Reps.

Volume has been identified as the likeliest single main driver of muscle growth. Each of the three variables—sets, reps and weight—increase volume. Therefore, increasing any one of those provides more stimulus to the muscles. However, if you play around with the numbers, it doesn't take long to realize that adding sets is the easiest way to significantly increase volume.

You can only increase the number of reps at a given weight so fast. And you can only increase the weight for a given number of reps so fast. But, it is relatively easy to add an extra set to any particular exercise. The only downside to this is that it adds more time to any given workout.

Adding more time to your workout is inconvenient. But more, it can be counter-productive. The more sets you pile into a single workout session, the less effort you are able to bring to the table on each set. Can you lift as much weight on set number 5 of an exercise than on set number one? How about on exercise number five? Certainly, the amount of effort you are able to generate for sets and exercises later in your routine is considerably less than the intensity you can generate in the first ones.

This point is obvious—you tire out as you do your workout. So what? Well, again remember there is a certain intensity below which muscle protein synthesis is simply not triggered. There is actually a new technical term in exercise science referring to this phenomenon: junk volume. "Junk Volume": refers to extra volume added to a workout which falls short of the threshold necessary to trigger muscle protein synthesis. It is wasted effort—it's like busy work in school. It just wastes your time to no purpose.

Because I coach Christian parents who have very little free time to fritter away, it is important to me that every single minute of their exercise time has meaning and contributes to attaining their physique goals. It is important to me that these aMPS be limited to 15 minutes in order to fit into the real lives of busy families. Thus, it becomes necessary to reduce the amount of rest between sets as the number of sets increases.

This too has its limits. If I want to keep the intensity level high and avoid the 15 minute session turning into a lower level of effort cardio session of continuous activity, there must be sufficient rest between sets to be able to give the necessary level of effort to each one. In general, I advocate resting enough to completely catch your breath between sets. I want the limiting factor of each set to be the targeted muscle group—not your cardiovascular capacity.

As one becomes acclimated to the workout regimen, one's general conditioning improves to support somewhat shorter rest periods; so I am able to progressively reduce the amount of rest between straight sets from an initial time of two minutes down to 90 seconds and again down to about 60 seconds. It then becomes necessary to introduce certain intensity techniques to be able to continue progressing the workout within the 15-minute time frame.

Myo-Reps

The intensity technique I incorporate into all client programs after they have maxed out exercise frequency, achieved a sufficient level of effort, and crammed as many sets as possible into a 15-minute workout, is a technique called myo-reps. Myo-reps rely upon an exercise science theory called "effective reps" theory. The theory of effective reps states that in any given set it is only the last five or six reps which really provide the mechanical tension challenge that stimulates muscle growth.

Think about it. If you do a set of 20 reps for an exercise, how challenging are those first 10 reps? They're pretty easy, right? In fact, at that point in the set you probably feel like you could go all day. It's only the last 5 or 6 reps that start feeling hard. Those first 10 or 15 were really just warm-up; they really just serve to tire you out to where the last 5 reps are challenging at all. Effective Reps theory would only count the last 5 reps of that 20 rep set. Even though you banged out 20 reps, only 5 did anything to stimulate muscle growth, the last 5.

Myo-reps capitalize on this scheme. You begin with a fairly light weight that you can get 20 reps with. In a normal straight set, you would do those 20 reps, rest for a minute or two, and then try to do 20 more. Then you might rest again before a third set and get 20 more. In Effective Reps theory, we count those 3 x 20 rep sets as a total of 15 "effective reps", the last 5 reps of each of those 3 sets.

Myo-reps begins with an "activation set" of 20 reps. But then, instead of resting two minutes and getting another set of 20, you only rest about 10 seconds, and then try to get five or six more reps. These five or six more reps are very challenging due to the short rest you just took. After that second set of five reps, you would rest ten seconds again, and then get another five reps. That whole cluster of three sets within that myo-reps exercise probably took about 90 seconds to do. Effective Reps theory would count that as 15 "effective reps", the same number of effective reps as you got in the previous example with straight sets. However, this took you 90 seconds to do whereas three straight sets took you 5 minutes. You get much more work done in much less time utilizing myo-reps.

There are other, more advanced intensity techniques that I might introduce into individual clients' programs when needed—techniques like drop sets or even occlusion training. However, for 95% of the people reading this book, a solid exercise progression would follow this pattern: 1) frequency, 2) intensity, or level of effort, 3) adding sets and reducing rest, and 4) myo-reps.

These aMPS are all of the exercise stimulus needed to trigger muscle protein synthesis and keep our bodies in a muscle-building state and out of a fat-storage state.

For a sample workout that shows one way to incorporate these principles into a concrete routine, see the resources section appended at the end of this book.

Dietary Support

Is exercise enough? Well, if we think about what we're trying to achieve, building muscle tissue, then the answer is no. Exercise is simply the event that stimulates the body process which follows. Specifically, aMPS stimulate muscle protein synthesis. Muscle protein synthesis is the bodily process which converts protein that we eat into protein that we wear, skeletal muscle tissue. It's clear from this recognition that we need the raw materials coming into our body before we can build muscle.

In the absence of sufficient protein through dietary intake, it's like trying to build a brick house without bricks. I don't care how skilled you are in construction; I don't care how much you know about designing homes; you simply cannot build a brick home without bricks. Neither can you build muscle without protein. So, the bare minimum dietary support for building muscle is adequate dietary protein intake.

It makes no sense to exercise without providing the dietary support necessary to achieve the goals of that exercise. If we are making the effort to stimulate muscle protein synthesis, then our diets must provide the basic building blocks necessary to achieve the results of muscle protein synthesis. Therefore, we always advocate a relatively high protein diet. How much is enough? Because everyone who follows this program will need to calculate their daily protein target, I included that discussion and methodology in the Action section in Week Four's lesson on protein.

What about carbs and fat?

Carbs and fat really serve a more limited purpose

inside the body. Each of them largely is just a source of energy. A such, they are interchangeable to a certain extent. While it is true that a certain amount of fat is essential in your diet, that amount is very small. It is such a small amount that it is almost impossible not to take in enough fat just as a by-product of all the other food that you eat. If you are incredibly vigilant on rooting out fats from your diet, you could theoretically end up with a shortfall of dietary fat. So, avoid restricting all fat from your diet. For 98% of the people reading this book, that will never be an issue. You have to be a superfood Nazi to cut out fat so drastically that you end up with a deficiency.

How about carbs? The fad diet marketing gurus would have you believe that carbs were manufactured by the devil to lead people into obesity and disease. This is exaggeration and oversimplification. What's the issue with carbs? If you have read all the marketing materials from the fad diet mills, I'm sure you have heard much to do about insulin sensitivity, insulin resistance and insulin response. Basically, it works like this.

When you eat carbs—any type of carbs, whether simple or complex—they are broken down by your body into units of simple sugar called glucose. These glucose molecules are carried in your bloodstream to all of your many cells that need a source of energy. Glucose is the body's preferred source of energy. To shuttle the glucose molecules from your bloodstream and into your cells requires insulin. Insulin is like a little key that unlocks the doors to the cells so that glucose can pass into them. This is how a healthy body works.

A problem can arise when you overeat carbs. Then, instead of merely having enough glucose in your blood to satisfy your cells' requirements for energy, you end up with too much glucose—more than your body can use. The more glucose that's in your blood at any one time, the more insulin is released by your pancreas in order to move that glucose into your cells. Thus, you end up with a ton of glucose and a ton of insulin in your bloodstream.

Just like a drug addict builds up a tolerance to any particular substance they are abusing, your cells also build up a tolerance to elevated levels of insulin. They start needing a higher dosage of insulin in order to open up their doors to transport glucose. This is called insulin resistance. Your cells stop responding to normal levels of insulin and require much higher levels. So what? Well, your pancreas can only produce so much insulin. At a certain point your cells require more insulin than your pancreas can supply. This is a condition called type two diabetes, and at this point you have to start supplying insulin from outside your body, from the pharmacy. So, eating too many carbs over a prolonged period can indeed have serious deleterious health effects.

Does that mean that carbs are evil? No. It's just like with anything else: The dose is the poison. Too much of any good thing stops being a good thing. Even water can kill you if you over-consume it. We need to moderate our carbohydrate intake. We don't necessarily need to avoid carbs all together, but most people who are in an over-fat condition are at risk for the situation described above. While the causal sequence can certainly be argued (whether insulin resistance causes fat gain or weather overeating and being over-fat cause insulin resistance), it's a chicken or the egg scenario which we can debate all day theoretically OR which we can address practically.

The practical cure in almost every instance is to lower body fat levels and moderate carbohydrate intake. We will lower body fat levels over the long-term by building muscle and allowing that to raise our resting metabolic rate, and we will eat a high protein diet which will replace much of the fat and carbohydrate intake to which we are accustomed.

If we eat a high protein diet and couple it with an appropriate calorie target, carbohydrate and fat levels will take care of themselves. This approach will not only be much easier to implement than micromanaging and counting every single carb, net carb, or fat gram; it will be more effective by supporting our goal of building muscle for the purpose of getting lean forever.

In the fad diet circles, beyond all the hubbub about insulin, you may even have heard about leptin and ghrelin, luteinizing hormone and follicle stimulating hormone, or HCG. These, though fascinating, are beyond the scope of this book. It is not that they are not interesting. They all are. It's just that they are not practical foci for your attention. They are fun to learn about, but focusing on any one of them is simply not worth your time in terms of action or results— theoretically interesting, but practically useless.

All of these rabbit trails are just that—rabbit trails. They are interesting, and there are loads of people who want a magic pill or effortless supplement that will make up for an unhealthy lifestyle, lack of exercise and poor diet. Heck, this includes 95% of the American healthcare practice (medicating symptoms). All these approaches focus on downstream symptoms rather than address the upstream cause of those symptoms.

It's like mobilizing a bunch of boats and machinery and

manpower to clean up sewage in a river. They launch a thousand boats and organize a huge, expensive operation to contain and clean up one patch after another of raw sewage waste. But, they don't venture upriver to confront the plant actually leaking sewage into the river. This makes no sense to me. Fix the source of the pollution, and the river is no longer being fouled in the first place! My main message is that we have come a long way in developing ways to fix the leaking sewage plants (unhealthy bodies) without having to spend hours in the gym, having to starve ourselves, or having to completely overhaul our lives.

Body Recomposition

In the section above, we talked about the necessity of a high protein intake to support muscle protein synthesis, which builds muscle, which raises our resting metabolic rate, which turns us into calorie-burning machines for life. But, if you are someone who is not currently at a high level of athletic fitness, then you are in a unique position to be able to do something that athletes normally cannot do: Body Recomposition.

Body Recomposition is a term that means gaining muscle and losing fat at the same time. It is pretty much the Holy Grail of all people seeking body transformation. The problem is, once you achieve a high level of physical fitness, it becomes almost impossible. Muscle is most easily built when you are eating an excess of calories. The absolute condition for losing fat is eating fewer calories then you expend. Thus, as you can see, the dietary requirements for both of those purposes are exact opposites. However...

When you are not in a state of athletic physical fitness, you can definitely build muscle while in a slight caloric deficit. As long as you are taking in enough protein, your body can dip into your own fat stores to supply the energy needed to fuel bodily activity and muscle protein synthesis—the muscle building process. And think about it, that is exactly what we want! We want to build muscle for our long-term leanness, and we want to use the energy stored in our body fat to supply the energy needs of our body. This is a total win-win scenario. And, it is a golden opportunity for someone who is out of shape to get a bigger bang for their buck, to double the return on their investment in terms of time and effort.

If you are out of shape right now, you can build muscle and burn fat at the same time. The reason this golden opportunity is not available to the same extent for people who are at a high level of physical fitness is because the body seeks a certain equilibrium. If you have a bunch of muscle on your frame right now, it takes a lot more concentrated effort to increase that. If you are extremely lean right now, is going to take a lot of very concentrated effort to get even leaner.

Your body seeks equilibrium. The further you are away from a "normal state", the easier it is to move towards that normal state, but the harder it is to move further away. The person who has a hundred pounds to lose will have an easier time losing 20 pounds than a person who only has 30 pounds to lose. They are further away from the "normal state". By the same token, the man who has built 50 extra pounds of muscle on his frame will have a much harder time putting on another 10 than the man who is malnourished. He is further away from the normal state and attempting to move to even greater extremes.

The body likes homeostasis. It likes equilibrium. It doesn't like to change. And it will usually, by default, move towards the normal state. Anyway, if you are extremely physically fit, if you are a practicing athlete with many months of consistent exercise and diet behind you, then it would be best to separate dedicated muscle-building phases from dedicated fat-loss phases. If, on the other hand, you are not currently at a high level of physical fitness, this opportunity for body recomposition—to gain muscle and lose fat at the same time—is a rare and golden opportunity lying right before you, literally begging you to reach out and take it. Here's how to do that.

JONAS & JACKIE SCHWARTZ

Sine-Wave Diet™

As we have discussed, diets, if they work, all boil down to one thing—calories in vs calories out. It doesn't matter if it is Paleo, South Beach, Keto, Low-fat, Low-carb, whatever. If it facilitates weight loss, it is about restricting calories. That's because calories are simply units of measurement (like inches) which measure the amount of energy you put in your body. So, when you hear "calories", think "energy".

Your overall energy balance determines whether you are gaining or losing fat. If you take in more energy (calories) than you expend, your body will store that energy for hard times in the form of body fat. Remember, our bodies' first goal is continued survival. Our DNA is not terribly worried about how we look in a bathing suit.

But we are...and our bodies are now facing a threat they have never faced before. In this day and age of cheap, plentiful food, the new health threat looming for most is actually obesity by overeating rather than death by starvation. We have to intentionally guide our bodies toward NOT storing a bunch of energy in the form of fat or else risk all the life-threatening diseases associated with obesity.

We have already decided we will address the calorie balance primarily through diet—as exercise is terribly inefficient in terms of calorie expenditure per minute. You can dedicate two hours of your day to a life-sapping treadmill OR you can decide NOT to eat a peanut butter sandwich. The choice is yours. For me, I'm going to reclaim my two hours I gave away, and just choose NOT to eat the sandwich.

That leaves diet to create a caloric deficit. That's why we developed an approach we call the Sine Wave™ Diet. The Sine Wave diet makes creating a caloric deficit as pain-free and productive as possible. This diet model simply allows for ups and downs in daily caloric intake. You do not have to meet a calorie target every single day. Instead, what is important is your calorie average over the week. Thus, if you overeat one day, you can make up for it over the next day or two. Or, if you have a big family meal every Sunday, you can eat a little lighter in the days leading up to it.

You must first determine your daily caloric target. That is of course easier said than done. The most accurate way to determine your daily caloric needs is to track your food intake overtime and plot that against your weight. After about a month of tracking every single thing that goes in your mouth, and keeping count of your calories, while weighing every day, you will get a pretty good idea of what daily calorie number causes you to gain weight and what daily caloric intake causes you to lose weight. The daily caloric intake where your weight does not move, where it stays the same over time, is called your maintenance calorie level.

Tracking over time is the most accurate way to find your maintenance calorie level. But, there are equations out there and calculators that allow you to get a decent ballpark estimate from which to start. If you Google "RMR" or "calorie" calculators, search results will fill your screen. These calculators use several different equations, but the most advanced is the Mifflin-St Jeor equation. Now remember, this is an estimate of your maintenance calories. It will not be absolutely accurate for anyone, but it is a decent ballpark guess for everyone. If you don't have the data above, several weeks worth of food tracking plotted against your body weight, then these calculators give you a good place to start. From there, you can begin tracking your food, tracking your weight and finding your maintenance calorie level.

Your maintenance calorie level is the number of calories you can eat per day and expect to maintain your weight, neither lose nor gained pounds. Obviously, if our goal is washing off body fat, we will need to eat less than this maintenance calorie level in order to create a caloric deficit. The common consensus is that it takes about a 500 calorie daily caloric deficit in order to lose a pound of body fat per week. You can be more or less aggressive in the rate at which you seek to lose body fat, but two pounds a week is about the maximum recommended by the scientific literature. So, we need to create anywhere between a 500-1000 calorie deficit in order to lose fat at the rate of one to two pounds per week. Thus, take your maintenance calorie level and subtract 500 to 1000 calories from it and make that your calorie target. That's a good place to start.

Here is where the Sine-Wave diet comes in. At this point, most coaches would tell you to hit your calorie target every single day, right on target every day. If you have ever tried to diet before while counting calories, you have probably experienced a bad day, a day when the numbers just did not add up the way you wanted them to. And then what happened? If you are like thousands of others, you probably got discouraged and gave up. And here's the crazy part: That is totally the wrong reaction because it is based upon a false assumption, the assumption that there is some magical 24-hour cut off period wherein success or failure is judged. That's crazy. Who said that?

There is no 24-hour period written into your body that determines how much fat you burn. A much more accurate guide for the amount of fat you will burn over time is a weekly average of your daily caloric intake. If you go over by a couple hundred calories on one day, then just make up for it on another. All we look at in our clients is the average at the end of the week. That is the only number we look for in terms of calories with our clients, and we have a 100% success rate for weight loss and body recomposition. This allows for a diet that fits real life!

Try to meet that goal as close as you can over the week. For instance, if your calorie goal is 1600 calories per day. Eating 1800 one day and 1400 another is perfectly fine. So is eating 2200 calories one day and 1500 the other six days. All we care about is the weekly average. That's why we call it the Sine Wave diet. It does not have to be linear—it can "Wave" up and down.

Imagine. You know you have a big family gathering on Sunday, and you know there will be all kinds of wonderful foods available. Why not just eat 100 calories less each day leading up to Sunday so that you can eat an extra 500 or 600 calories of all the delicious food? If the outcome is the same in terms of fat loss, why would you not do that?

If you decide to go out and eat this evening with your family, but you don't have the calories left in your daily budget to eat anything at the restaurant, do you just tell your family, "Sorry I can't go?" No. Go eat with your family. If you go over your calorie goal by a few hundred calories today, just tighten your belt and make up for it over the next few days. No harm no foul. Your diet is still on track. It's not broken at all. You get to live like a real person, and you have a sustainable diet model that you can keep up over the few weeks that it takes to execute a dietary intervention.

This is one of the most popular features of our program with our clients, the flexibility to allow for variations in calorie levels throughout the week. As long as your average calorie intake is close to your goal, then what's the problem? Our clients don't have a problem, and they consistently gain muscle and lose fat on our 12-week program, every time.

Now, just like with resistance training exercise, there has to be a sort of progression built into the diet model as well. The body is remarkably adaptive, and every time you drop calories, your body will attempt to adapt and function at that lower calorie level. When this happens, when you cease to see a new low weight on the scale for an entire week, you will need to drop calories again. These subsequent drops, after that initial 500 to a thousand calorie drop, are much smaller in scale. We're talking about 150 to 200 calories. Whenever a week goes by without you seeing a new low on the scale, it's time to implement one of these small drops. Thus, just like with adding challenge to your exercises in order to force your muscles to adapt, we have to continue to add challenges in caloric intake to force your body to tap into its fat stores to supplement the caloric deficit. Your body was built and designed not to starve. It's pretty good at surviving low-calorie periods of time.

So, there is a limited window of time during which we can effectively diet for fat-loss. This is because there is a minimum calorie threshold that you need to eat in order to keep up basic bodily functions. This is probably somewhere between 800 and 1200 calories, depending on your body size. And this minimum number of calories is not a place you want to live long term. It is a place you want to briefly visit at the very end of a multiple week diet. For instance, if you are dieting for eight weeks, then hopefully this basement level of calories will not be necessary until you are five or six weeks or into the diet. Then you only have to grind out a couple of weeks at this very low-calorie level. It is not healthy to stay there for long.

So, what then?

Cycling

A fat-loss diet is an intervention; it is a short-term treatment for a specific condition. That condition is obesity, or being over-fat. A fat-loss diet is a temporary treatment. It is not meant to be the way that you live forever. It is merely a corrective treatment. That doesn't mean you can't learn some healthier eating habits while you are employing the intervention, but you should not live on a low-calorie diet for life. It's unhealthy, and scientifically speaking, that would totally suck.

The research shows that the most effective length of time for fat-loss diets are anywhere from 6 to 12 weeks. If you do some quick math, with the rate of fat loss that we outlined above, 1 to 2 pounds a week, you can quickly see that most of these diets result in a loss of 10 to 20 pounds of body fat during that time. What if you have more than that to lose?

Here's what most people do—and why they either fail altogether or quickly regain their weight. They usually continue at extremely low calorie levels. Or, perhaps they add more hours to their cardio regimens. I can't tell you how many clients we have had come into our program eating 900 or fewer calories a day and spending two to three hours doing low cardio programs daily. And guess what? Even at these extremes, they have ceased to lose weight.

The answer is really very simple. It's not obvious, but it is simple. They have dieted for so long, and they have worked their bodies so many hours for so long, that they are in a very unhealthy, run-down state. The prolonged low-calorie diet has absolutely crashed their metabolisms as well as their hormone levels. People are literally in starvation mode.

Their bodies are preserving every last little bit of body tissue that they can. Their cortisone levels (the stress hormone) is through the roof, and their thyroid levels (which to a large extent regulate metabolism) are absolutely bottomed out. If a physician gave them a blood test right now, they would be shocked at the shape they are in.

Metabolic Priming™

The first thing we have to do with clients who come into the program in this condition, is to feed them and heal them. We call this Metabolic Priming™. We have to slowly raise their calories back to a normal maintenance state and dial back their exercises to a level that their bodies can recover from. They're starving and overtrained. (See the discussion above on metabolic adaptation). Is there anything worse than exercising for hours every day and literally starving yourself while getting absolutely no results for your suffering? You wouldn't believe how common this is.

This is one segment of the population that the current health and fitness and diet gurus love to target and prey upon. These are people actively engaged in dieting and exercise, who are interested in both, who have shown that interest by following some sort of structured diet and exercise program, and who have ceased to see results from their efforts. What better market is there than a bunch of sweaty, starving people who are utterly frustrated with all the time, work, and suffering they are putting in day after day to no avail?

So, the normal marketing approach from mainstream, popular snake-oil salesman is to focus on these current symptoms that are a result of a crashed metabolism. They focus on the insulin response which is out of whack due to a prolonged starvation diet. They focus on hormonal imbalances, which are all direct results of a prolonged starvation diet. They focus on products and stimulants that can marginally boost caloric expenditure (like caffeine) in order to address the slowed, sluggish metabolism which is a direct result of a prolonged starvation diet.

Look guys, this is utterly shortsighted. It's profitable for the snake-oil salesman, but these are tiny little rabbit trails which are unnecessary and not worth your time to explore. Every one of those symptoms listed was a result of a prolonged starvation diet. The solution is not to address each individual symptom in a pointless effort to remedy that particular symptom. No, the solution is to address the underlying problem which causes all of those downstream symptoms in the first place.

Honestly, the fad diet industry is simply following the methodology of our health care system when they do this. Our health care system is very quick to prescribe all sorts of expensive and dangerous pharmaceuticals to alleviate particular symptoms, but it's very rare that you get any sort of meaningful help from your doctor to address the CAUSE of all those symptoms—being in an overall state of ill health—far from your ideal body weight, and a perfect candidate for all of the diseases for which they are very happy to prescribe you medicines.

As I've previously stated, my thinking is that we should focus on the cause of all these symptoms rather than chase down every individual effect—go for the root of the problem, move ourselves from a state of ill health to health, and then see what symptoms persist from there. Usually that takes care of pretty much everything. The body is remarkable in its capacity to heal itself when everything is working in balance and in order as it was designed to work. When the different systems of your body are out of balance and out of whack, that's when we are at risk for all of those obesity-related illnesses we are so familiar with: Diabetes, hypertension, stroke, and heart attacks. It's no wonder the new epidemic in America is obesity.

So, the last thing that you want to do when you get to the end of a 6 to 12 week diet is to mindlessly continue at a very low calorie level for an extended period of time. No, you have to give your body a break. We aim to reduce body fat by about 10% each dietary cycle. After losing 10 to 20 pounds of fat over an 8 to 10 week diet, you need to reverse diet—slowly raise your calories back up to maintenance levels in order to allow your body to recover, heal and prepare for the next dietary cycle.

Remember to reverse diet, though. Do not instantly jump back to your former maintenance calorie level, or you will pile some fat back on. You must raise your calories slowly over the course of a few weeks and then stay at a good, healthy maintenance level for about another four weeks. Then, your metabolism will be revved up, your hormones will be back in balance, and you will be ready to go another round on the diet, and lose another 10% of your body fat.

Now, you could look at this time outside of your fat-loss diet as wasted time. Nobody likes wasted time! But remember, our overall strategy for long-term fat loss is to build muscle. Guess what? That low calorie diet that we just came out of has put our bodies into the perfect position to gain a good bit of muscle during our short diet break. This too is a golden opportunity. You use these maintenance periods to build up muscle tissue and then you use the low-calorie diet periods to wash off body fat.

The two cycles complement each other perfectly and set one another up perfectly. It is a match made in heaven, and it is no wonder that physique athletes have used exactly this iterative cycle for gaining muscle and losing body fat for years. No bodybuilders have achieved their level of muscularity and leanness by staying at one calorie level constantly over time. No. Rather, they cycle over and over and over again, every time gaining a little bit more muscle and losing a little bit more fat. Over the course of a few cycles, you have literally transformed your body forever.

This is psychologically refreshing too. Think about it, at the end of a 12-week diet, you are dreaming of all the food that you have deprived yourself of over the past two or three months. Guess what? Within a couple of weeks, you'll be eating them again, pizza and all.

Those four weeks at maintenance will be like an oasis in the desert. And, you will be able to stick to your low calorie diet better at the end, knowing that it is only temporary—that if you just make it a couple more weeks, you'll be eating pizza and ice cream. I don't want it to sound like I eat nothing but junk food, because I don't. But the point is when you are on your maintenance period, you are building muscle. You have far more freedom to fit far more foods into your daily caloric intake than you can when you are in the low-calorie fat-loss period.

There is a time and a season for everything. Embrace where you are in the cycle and enjoy it. This does not have to be a soul-crushing, life-draining experience. Rather, let it be a source of joy and reaffirm your vitality and joy in life!

Recovery

No discussion of the workout, exercise or muscle-building process is complete without a thorough consideration of recovery. Together with exercise and diet, recovery completes the three pillars of success in terms of body composition change. If you neglect any one of these components, your progress will be slowed, stopped or even reversed depending on how severely the principles are violated.

"Exercise" in our context means one thing and one thing only—presenting a stimulus adequate to elicit the response we want, building muscle. It is the muscle we build which burns away our excess body fat, not the blood, sweat and tears we cry in the gym. Thus, as long as the stimulus meets the minimum threshold of "flipping the switch" to activate Muscle Protein Stimulus, the stimulus is adequate to meet our goals.

But what if we did more exercise than was necessary? Or, what if besides stimulating Muscle Protein Synthesis we also added in a variety of physical activity in our quest to burn fat?

This is tricky. This is where the consideration of recovery comes into play. But when we say "recovery", what do we really mean? Recovery is simply our ability to respond to a stressor, and any kind of physical activity is indeed a stressor. It stresses the body.

Understand, however, that our ability to respond to stressors is limited. If you have ever helped someone move lots of furniture or engaged in marathon workout sessions or been in a car accident, you introduced a large amount of stress on your body. It probably took you days to recover and heal up. These sorts of things are further along the continuum of stressors—more like injuries. But what we need to understand here is that any sorts of physical activity introduce stress on the body and require time, sleep and nutrition in order to recover.

In terms of exercise, there is a well-documented phenomenon called "over-training". This refers to the act of presenting more stress (through exercise) than your body can recover from in a timely manner. If you overtrain regularly, your body will actually become more and more depleted, tired and in some cases injured. Think about that. You are trying to build up your health, but you can actually break yourself down by overtraining. Like many other things in life, while exercise is good, too much of a good thing can be bad.

So, the question is how do we balance our limited recovery ability with our exercise efforts? How do we manage it? The answer lies in thinking of exercise as a medicine. We need to prescribe a dosage, an amount that is effective without being harmful (even Tylenol is deadly if you dose too high).

The 15 minute aMPS workouts are designed precisely to provide an adequate stimulus while staying far from an excessive dose. Effective NOT Excessive. I don't know about you, but I want to do just enough to be confident I am presenting an adequate stimulus, with equal confidence that I am not wasting time doing more exercise than necessary--which might actually be tearing down the body I am trying to build up!

This is why I do not advocate doing things like Camp Gladiator or Crossfit while trying to change your body. I have made the argument that building muscle is the most rational way to lose fat (see above argument about raising Resting Metabolic Rate). Thus, if I am trying to change my body, I need to SPECIFICALLY TARGET building muscle as my goal and pursue it with single-minded focus. Muscle is built by stimulating Muscle Protein Synthesis. ANYTHING I do that does not bring about that end is taking me away from my goal.

The research is crystal clear. Progressive resistance strength training is the most effective means of building muscle. Running laps does not do it. Doing mountain climbers, burpees and bear crawls doesn't do it. Rowing, biking, swimming don't do it in anywhere near as effective a manner as progressive resistance strength training. Thus, while my focus is on changing my body composition (losing fat and gaining muscle), I am best served by a single-minded focus on my goal. All those other activities eat into my recovery abilities. By themselves, they don't build muscle, and added on to progressive resistance strength training, they constitute added stressors which may prove too much for my ability to recover.

If you ENJOY these activities, I am not saying give them up for life. But WHILE you are concentrating on changing your body composition, while you are trying to lose fat and gain muscle, put them on hold. Come back to them once you have established a healthy body fat percentage at which you are comfortable. Then, enjoy! Until then, focus on what actually works to change your body for good.

PART II

15 MINUTE FAT LOSS FORMULA

CHAPTER 4
COMMITMENTS & STRUCTURE

My wife Jackie and I have tested and optimized the following twelve-week program to use with our clients. It is intentionally simple, as no matter how excellent and well-designed a diet and exercise program may be, it is absolutely worthless if it can't fit into the life of the client seeking to implement it. The greatest tool in the world is useless if it is too difficult to wield.

Thus, we break down every step of this progress program into a series of 12 weekly challenges which focus on one thing and one thing only. Week by week, we build upon the foundation laid in the previous week so that by the end of week twelve, you have created a marvelous structure.

We don't want to overwhelm you with information, directives and assignments to the point where something gets left by the wayside. I need you to master each one of these topics in order, because they are presented in order of importance. The things at the beginning are more important than the things at the end. Therefore, take your time, truly make the effort to make the meet each particular week's challenge so that it becomes a habit in your life before moving on. While it is true that a reduced calorie diet is meant to be temporary and not lifelong, the principles that you will learn throughout this program can be used continually the rest of your life. If you have mastered them, you will always have those valuable tools in your toolbox to use at the appropriate times.

So, let's get started!

Commitments & Structure

In order to best guide you through these 12 weeks of fat-loss and muscle-building, you will need data. The better data you keep, the better tweaks you can make to your program, and the better your results will be.

Commitments...We need 2 commitments from the beginning:

1)   WEIGH YOURSELF EVERY DAY AND LOG IT. We use an app called Cronometer, and we use the professional version to coach all our clients. There is a free version as well, and we highly recommend it. Your body weight fluctuates daily due to fluctuations in water weight. But, you need as many data points as possible so you will be able to discern the overall trend AS IT IS BEING ESTABLISHED. So, as soon as you get out of bed, use the toilet and then weigh--every day.

2)   LOG EVERYTHING YOU EAT. Again, we use and recommend Cronometer. Logging food is a pain. It is. I know. But, it is the most accurate way to keep tabs on your nutrition. I promise I will NEVER waste your time (we are the home of the 15 minute workout, remember), but logging food is worth the effort.

There is a learning curve, and you will not become expert at it overnight (or in a week or two). But it will get easier and faster as you get accustomed to it, and the app learns the foods you habitually eat. Over these 12 weeks, you will get better and better--giving yourself better and better data to base your decisions upon. And you will learn more about how your body responds to different foods than you ever knew before. Search YouTube for Cronometer tutorials if you want a video guide to get started. We have links to good ones in our

Facebook group, "Fit Families of Faith" and on our YouTube channel: "15minute.fitness".

Chronological Structure

Phase I: Metabolic Priming (2-4 weeks)

This is the set-up for the diet that follows. We want to rev up our metabolisms and build a base of strength before we begin trying to lose fat. Failure to properly set up a diet is very often the reason diets fail.

Phase II: Diet-Intensity (2-4 weeks)

Here we "push start" the fat loss process. The whole object is to get the ball rolling, breaking through to new lows and establishing a down trend on the scale.

Phase III: Diet-Duration (4-8 weeks)

This is where we make adjustments as necessary to keep the ball rolling as far and as fast as it will go.

CHAPTER 5
PHASE 1—METABOLIC PRIMING

Setting up Training

If you bought a copy of this book, then I will give you 30 day access to my free beginner's workout program on the training app we use with our paid clients, "15minute.fitness". Just go to www.15minute.fitness and sign up for our "Free Foundations Course." It is a 1 page course that explains our basic approach. At the end of that page, you'll find the offer for free app access.

Too many people fail in their health and fitness pursuits due to lack of preparation. Taking the little time necessary to lay solid foundations makes all the difference. Our clients who have followed that 1 page course have shown exponentially better results than those who choose not to.

Setting up the diet, self-diagnosis

The first phase of the diet is Metabolic Priming. Metabolic Priming is our term for laying the groundwork for a successful diet. It is preparation (priming the pump) for the diet phases which follow.

Everyone enters into the program from a unique set of circumstances. Some will come into this program having overfed themselves for years. The first step in metabolic priming for these is to introduce daily, muscle-building workouts to move them into a state of muscle-building rather than fat-storage. We want their bodies to get accustomed to shuttling excess calories toward muscle tissue rather than body fat.

On the other hand, if you remember, we talked about the too common phenomenon of someone eating so few calories or exercising so much that they have essentially crashed their metabolism. Their hormone levels are at terribly unhealthy marks, and they have ceased being able to lose weight no matter how few calories they eat or how much they exercise. Metabolic Priming for these takes the form of a full-scale Metabolic Reboot™ (a longer, more intensive metabolic priming). Along with appropriate, moderate levels of muscle-building exercises, we will introduce more calories into their daily intake in order to allow their bodies to heal, their metabolisms to be restored and their hormones to reestablish normal, balanced levels.

We can actually test for this condition during the first two to four weeks of our program and alleviate it. Here's how. For the first two weeks of the diet, everyone is directed to eat at their maintenance calorie level. Remember, this is the calorie level at which you neither gain nor lose weight. If you don't know your maintenance calorie level, then we calculate a baseline estimate and assign that to you as your target. We ask you to hit that calorie intake goal as closely as possible each day, with the built-in flexibility of the Sine Wave diet—more on that in week two—for the first two weeks. With those two weeks of data, your daily caloric intake and your daily body weight, we can make rational decisions about the next step in your diet process.

If, after eating at your maintenance level for two weeks, your weight is consistently moving downward, then we know that your body is used to eating more calories than that. You have been overeating in the past, and your weight is moving down because of the relative caloric deficit we have created. Believe it or not, this is the best-case scenario. The fix for it is simple, continue progressively reducing calories to keep you losing weight. We will label the group of you who fit into this category "Overeaters". Throughout the 12-week program outlined below, watch for special directives aimed at "Overeaters".

If, after eating at maintenance level for two weeks, your weight is not noticeably trending downwards or upwards, but rather moving sideways, staying about the same, then we will label your group "Maintainers". Our strategy for you, and the timing of caloric drops in your diet, will be different than for overeaters. Watch for special directives over the 12-week program aimed at "Maintainers".

Finally, if after eating at maintenance level for two weeks, your weight is moving upwards, that means you were not eating enough calories in the weeks or months before the program. You are in the category labeled "Undereaters", and you are in need of a full Metabolic Priming phase. We have to heal your rundown metabolism, rev it up, and re-balance your crashed hormone levels before we can successfully diet you down to reduce body fat. Thus, you can expect the first four weeks of the diet to having you eat more than you are accustomed to. Don't expect to lose body fat during the first 4 weeks. This is remedial work you have to do to put yourself into a position from which you can successfully diet.

Sometimes, it is emotionally difficult not to see weight loss over a four-week block of time, but I would encourage you to see this as a time of muscle-building and preparation. This is not idle time. This is vitally necessary in order to break through the plateau and drag yourself out of the hole that you have dug. Watch for your special directives aimed at "Undereaters" during the program.

We do this with our private coaching clients. However, as the VAST majority entering the program do turn out to need a metabolic reboot, we automatically begin our premium program group members with a full Metabolic Priming phase. It never hurts, and always helps, to tone and build muscle and to fully rev your metabolism before entering a full-blown diet phase. To simplify the program, I would suggest embracing that model by following the directives for "Undereaters" in the action steps below.

Set up: Calorie Target

Now is the time to set up Cronometer with your initial calorie target. If you have been tracking your food intake for several weeks and plotting it against your scale weight, then you will know your maintenance calorie level—the calorie count at which your weight neither rises nor falls. Plug this number into cronometer as your daily calorie target.

If you have not been tracking your food or you don't know your maintenance calorie level, you can get an estimate by using an online RMR Calculator. Do a Google search for "Mifflin-St Jeor RMR Calculator". This is the most recent version of an algorithm meant to estimate your daily caloric needs. The calculator you find will ask you for the inputs: Age, height, weight, gender, and activity level. Then it will spit out an estimate for you. Take this number and plug it into Cronometer as your daily calorie target. Try to eat as close as you can to that amount each day. It is a good guestimate to begin with.

You will also need a daily protein target. This will get more specific in Week Three. For now, simply plug in a number of grams of protein equal to your ideal body weight in pounds—what you would like to weigh. (If you think your ideal body weight is 150lbs, then eat 150 grams of protein per day). Eat that amount (or close to it) now. We'll get more precise in Week Three.

JONAS & JACKIE SCHWARTZ

WEEK 1
aMPS™: MUSCLE PROTEIN SYNTHESIS ACTIVATORS
&
SLEEP

Challenge:
Exercise—aMPS
Recovery—Sleep
(Theoretical Foundations p 43)

aMPS: The foundation of our program is a rational scientific approach to exercise—probably different from what you have experienced in the past. You have probably heard that you need to burn calories in your workout; after all, you have to burn more calories than you eat to lose weight. That's grade school physics.

Yes...BUT

It is FAR easier to address the calorie balance component through diet. If you want to run for 2 hours on a treadmill, so you can eat an extra peanut butter sandwich, by all means, don't let me stop you. Me? I'm just going to forego the peanut butter sandwich, and save my energy and time for the busy life I lead. Either option has the same effect on calorie balance. Exercise is pretty inefficient at burning calories. My day job and my family responsibilities don't allow for hour-long, marathon exercise sessions anyway.

For my exercise time, I want to accomplish ONE mission and one mission only: "flip the switch" to activate muscle protein synthesis. That directs the calories I eat over the next 24-48 hours toward building muscle instead of storing fat. And the muscle I build raises my Resting Metabolic Rate (RMR)—the amount of calories I burn day in and day out...at rest, literally while I do nothing more than breathe. The more muscle you have, the more calories you burn...simply existing.

The bonus for us as busy people with real lives is that we can activate muscle protein synthesis in properly designed 15 minute workouts. And the muscle-building signals we have initiated last for 24 hours-48 hours. Thus, 15 minute daily Muscle Protein Synthesis Activation workouts (aMPS) are all the exercise you need to radically transform your body over time, forever.

Extra bonus: While a two-hour workout will leave you drained the rest of the day (and likely the next day as well), a 15 minute workout really revs your metabolism and gets your juices flowing, GIVING you energy for the rest of your real life and family instead of sucking the life out of you. Win-Win!

Lesson:
Sleep

Sleep: Believe it or not, research shows adequate sleep is as important (if not more) in terms of muscle-gain and fat-loss as training and nutrition. Meditate on that a moment. Can you really get that big of a boost in body composition change from something that is totally easy—and that we actually LIKE to do? YES!

You like to sleep! I bet you don't leap out of bed when your alarm goes off. No. Our minds and bodies LIKE sleep; it is good for us! And it is easy—you don't have to sweat in a gym or choke down a ton of raw, leafy greens. All you have to do to MARKEDLY boost your results is sleep! Your target is 8 hours in bed, in sleep mode.

There are several things you can do to help improve your sleep.

1.   Take a melatonin supplement. Melatonin is a natural hormone released by your body as part of the diurnal cycle. It signals sleep time. Not only will it help you sleep, but it is also one of the most powerful antioxidants known to science. That alone is reason to use it. Start with five mg and slowly work up to 15 or 20 over time, if you can.

2.   Create a bedtime routine. As parents, we do this for our children. We give them a bath, we have them brush their teeth, we read them a story, we tuck them in and kiss them goodnight. This nightly routine trains our brain. It is a signal that we are slowing down and getting ready to sleep, and it is a signal for our brain to start relaxing our bodies and shutting down. It can be as simple as washing your face, brushing your teeth, putting on pajamas and spending a few minutes reading or winding down.

3.   Shut down the screens. Turn your electronics off at least 30 minutes before you want to fall asleep, an hour is even better. It takes your brain time to recover from the light emitted by our phones and computer screens and to settle down from information overload.

4.   Turn on white noise. You no longer have to buy a special device to get white noise while you sleep. There are a number of apps that you can put on your phone or tablet that will play a variety of white noise sounds. Who doesn't like to fall asleep to the sound of rain. It quiets the chatter of our own mind.

5.   Take a hot shower or bath 30 minutes to an hour before you want to sleep. As your body temperature cools off you will become more tired.

6.   Try essential oils. You can put oils into a diffuser or use a lotion that has oils known to help you relax and sleep. Lavender is always a winner.

7.   Have a snack. Now is the time for some carbs. What? Carbs!? Yes. Eating carbs causes your insulin to spike and as it falls you get sleepy. This is the cause of mid-day slump after a high carb breakfast. Use it to your advantage at nighttime.

For further information, we have videos on YouTube on the benefits of sleep plus tips to sleep better. Search for "Sleep" on our YouTube Channel, "15minute.fitness".

Weekly Challenge 1: aMPS Workouts and Sleep

aMPS: This week, I want to move towards making 15 minute daily training a habit. The first thing a recovering alcoholic is advised to do is attend 90 AA meetings in 90 days. This is so that it becomes a daily habit. Make your aMPS daily habits. (The default schedule is six aMPS per week with one day off). In our coaching and membership programs, clients access these workouts in our custom 15minute.fitness™ training app.

If you are doing this alone without membership to our program or personal coaching, find some way to track your workout regimen and your progress. There are apps available for your phone; you can make a spreadsheet; or, you can use good old-fashioned pencil and paper. The point is to have your exercise program accessible to you while working out, including the weights and reps you tracked from the previous week. Progressing over time is key.

Now, START LIGHT. These do not need to be hard workouts this week. Start slow and don't do any exercises that are painful or just don't feel right. This first week is dedicated to breaking you in on a muscle-building exercise regime. I don't need all-out effort here. Be kind to your body. We're focusing on habit right now, not intense effort. There is plenty of time to ramp up effort and intensity level later.

BONUS TIP: POST-WORKOUT REWARD!

There are no "evil" foods. Even straight pig lard can be good—for a starving person or an eskimo looking to add insulation and extra fuel to his reserves (body fat). It is all relative.

Right after your workout is THE PERFECT TIME for a SUGARY SNACK. Your body dipped into its glycogen stores during strength training, and replenishing those stores is a necessary part of the recovery process. You want to stay away from fat here, but sugar/starch and protein are absolute gold. We like low fat cupcakes (Jackie has a recipe) iced with a chocolate or cinnamon flavored protein powder glaze. Oh yeah. Or, I like kids cereal—cinnamon toast crunch is pretty awesome. If you have a sweet tooth, right after your workout is THE time to indulge it; It actually does your body good.

Sleep: 8 hours in bed, in sleep mode—not including time spent reading or winding-down. Sleep mode. Every Night.

TLDR: 6 workouts, 8 hours sleep each night

WEEK 2
SINE WAVE DIET™

Challenge:
Nutrition—Calories
(Theoretical Foundations p 67)

We already went into some depth on calories in the introductory sections, but as calories are the focal topic of Week Two, much of what was already said bears repeating. This is the week to absolutely master setting a calorie target and hitting it, at least in terms of weekly average. The following few paragraphs review what was already said, but this week you are not merely learning about the conceptual principles in thermodynamics behind the caloric model of energy expenditure and fat loss, you are actually implementing it. So, review the following paragraphs, and then we will outline a plan of action for you this week.

Diets, if they work, all boil down to one thing--calories in vs calories out. It doesn't matter if it is paleo, South Beach, Keto, low-fat, low-carb, whatever. If it facilitates weight loss, it is about restricting calories. That's because calories are simply units of measurement (like inches) which measure the amount of energy you put in your body. So, when you hear "calories", think "energy" and vice versa.

Your overall energy balance determines whether you are gaining or losing fat. If you take in more energy (calories) than you expend, your body will store that energy for hard times in the form of body fat. Remember, our bodies' first goal is continued survival. Our DNA is not terribly worried about how we look in a bathing suit.

But we are...and our bodies are now facing a threat they have never faced before. In this day and age of cheap, plentiful food, the new health threat looming for most is actually overeating rather than death by starvation. We have to intentionally guide our bodies toward NOT storing a bunch of energy in the form of fat or else risk all the life-threatening diseases associated with obesity. Last week, we decided we would address the calorie balance primarily through diet—as exercise is terribly inefficient in terms of calorie expenditure per minute. You can dedicate two hours of your day to running on a life-sapping treadmill OR you can decide to NOT eat a peanut butter sandwich. The choice is yours. For me, I'm going to reclaim my two hours I gave away, and just choose NOT to eat the peanut butter sandwich.

That leaves diet to create a caloric deficit. And for us, the "Sine Wave" diet makes this as pain free and productive as possible. The Sine Wave diet simply allows for ups and downs in daily caloric intake. You do not have to meet a calorie target every single day. Instead, what is important is your calorie average over the week. Thus, if you overeat one day, you can make up for it over the next day or two. Or, if you have a big family meal every Sunday, you can eat a little lighter in the days leading up to it.

This week, you need to determine a calorie goal. If you are following our recommendation, you will put this goal in Cronometer and log the food you eat in order to reach this goal. Try to meet that goal as closely as you can over the week. For instance, if your calorie goal is 1600 calories per day. Eating 1800 one day and 1400 another is perfectly fine. So is eating 2200 calories one day and 1500 the other six days. All we care about is the weekly average. That's why we call it the Sine Wave diet. It does not have to be linear—it can "Wave" up and down.

Weekly Challenge 2: Calories

1.   Make sure you have a daily calorie target. See the section called "Set-up: Calories" in the introduction portion of the Practice Section.

2.   Hit that calorie target in terms of **weekly average** from here on out!

WEEK 3
PROTEIN

Calorie Setup:

From this point on, we will include a "set-up" section before each weekly lesson. This will give you some numerical, behind-the-scenes directives needed to manipulate your calorie targets each week.

At this point, you have two weeks of data, daily calorie intake and daily body weight. If you have been consistently hitting your daily maintenance calorie intake, at least in terms of weekly average as explained in the section on the Sine Wave Diet from week two, then the only thing you need to examine is your weight over the last two weeks. Has it moved up or down at least two pounds?

When I say, "Track your weight," I need to give direction. I want you ONLY to note the low weight over the past seven days. Different bodies fluctuate different amounts daily due to water weight, but ALL bodies fluctuate in body weight daily. What I am referring to when I ask you to "track your weight" is your weekly low weight. So, right now, compare the low weight from week two to your low weight from week one. Is week two's low weight higher or lower than week one's low weight?

If it has moved up two pounds, label yourself an "Undereater" and follow directives for Undereaters from here on. If it has moved down two pounds, label yourself an "Overeater" and follow directives for Overeaters for the duration of the 12-week program. If it has stayed within 2 pounds of your starting weight, label yourself a "Maintainer" and follow those directives going forward.

Overeaters: drop your target calories by 100 for this week. You have now moved into Phase 2 of the diet.

Undereaters: You will need to remain in Phase 1 (Metabolic Priming) for another two weeks. Keep your target calories the same for the next two weeks in order to implement a Metabolic Reboot.

Maintainers: (Simple version) Drop your target calories by 400 calories for a woman and 700 calories for a man. You have now moved into Phase 2 of the diet.

Maintainers: (Complex version) Choose how aggressive you want to be on this diet. You can lose the same amount of weight in two different ways. You can reduce calories moderately over the course of 12 weeks or you can reduce calories more aggressively over the course of 6 to 8 weeks. This comes down to personal choice. Everyone's body responds slightly differently to moderate versus aggressive caloric reductions. And everyone has psychological preferences in terms of how long and how hard they want to diet. But, both methods usually result in very similar outcomes. Choose one now according to the numbers below.

Reduce your maintenance calorie total by 500 to 1000 calories depending on your choice above. Reduce it by 500 or so if you prefer a longer, milder diet. And reduce it by up to 1000 if you prefer a shorter, more aggressive diet. That said, there are a couple of more considerations to make before you choose your calorie deficit.

Because I never want a female below 800 calories or a male below 1200 calories, you have a built-in minimum number of calories. And because phase two of this program includes a feedback loop where you will continue to cut calories if your weight doesn't drop a certain amount each week, we can't get too close to our basement level calories just yet. Therefore, when you select your initial 500 to 1000 calorie drop, make sure your target number is not less than 1700 for a man or 1200 for a woman. That leaves us a little room for further tweaks later on throughout the 12-week program.

Challenge:
Nutrition—Protein
(Theoretical Foundations see below)

Explanation and Rationale
Behind calories, protein is the next biggest factor in your diet. Protein is necessary for tissue repair and muscle growth as well as providing the raw materials for hormones and enzymes. It also converts to energy if necessary, but does so inefficiently, which is a good thing for our purposes.

Research shows that consuming at least 20 grams of protein independently stimulates muscle protein synthesis. Remember that term? That's what we do when we do a muscle-building workout. So, eating 20 or more grams of protein in a meal is like getting a small mini-workout in.

However, research shows that we can't use more than around 40 to 50 grams of protein at one time. Therefore, it is important to space protein feedings out fairly evenly over the course of the day. So, you need to plan on eating four meals at a minimum each day, and each meal should have between 20-50 grams of protein. That's like getting an extra mini-workout in, 4 times a day! Now we're really ramping things up!

For further information, we have videos on YouTube on why protein is so important, as well as suggestions and tips to help you with your protein intake. Search for "Protein" on our YouTube Channel, "15minute.fitness".

Weekly Challenge 3: Protein

First, we have to calculate a specific daily protein target. The consensus of literature in the scientific community has coalesced around the figure of one gram of protein per pound of lean body weight for people trying to build muscle. A fairly simple rule of thumb that you can use is to imagine yourself at your ideal weight. Aim for about 1 gram of protein per pound of that ideal body weight per day. For instance, if you are a 6-foot tall man, and you imagine yourself at an ideal body weight of 185 pounds, then aim for 185 grams of protein per day while trying to build muscle. If, on the other hand, you are a five foot, two inch woman, and you imagine yourself at an ideal body weight of 125 pounds, then aim to take in 125 grams of protein per day while trying to build muscle. Are these exact numbers? No. But they are easy rules of thumb that gets you into the ballpark.

A more exact calculation would require us to factor in your target body fat percentage. We can use rough target estimates of 10% body fat for a man and 20% for a woman. You could then take those estimates we came up with and reduce them by 10% or 20% respectively. Thus, a more accurate target for the 6-foot man who wants to weigh 185 pounds would come out to be about 165 grams of protein per day (185 * .9). while the more exact estimate for the 5'2" woman who wants to weigh 125 pounds would be 100 grams of protein per day (125*.8). These would be the protein targets we would assign to our clients in our coaching program.

So, imagine yourself at your ideal weight. Take that number and multiply by .9 (for a man) or .8 (for a woman). That is now your protein goal in grams per day. Plug that number in Cronometer, and eat that amount of protein each day, spaced out fairly evenly over 4 or more meals. For instance, if your daily target is 160g protein, spread that over 4 meals with about 40g each.

WEEK 4
FIBER & HYDRATION

Calorie Setup:

Overeaters & Maintainers: Did you hit a new low weight during this last week that was at least one pound lower than your low weight from the week before? If the answer is yes, then leave your calories the same this week. If the answer is no, then reduce your calories by 150 for a woman or 200 for a man. Remember, never reduce your calories below 800 for a woman or 1200 for a man under any circumstances. You will continue this feedback loop until Week Ten.

Undereaters: This is the last week of your Metabolic Reboot; calories remain the same. Your first drop will be at the beginning of Week Five. By that time, your metabolism should be revved up, and your body should be healed up enough to sustain and succeed with an 8-week diet.

Challenge:
Nutrition—Fiber & Hydration
(Theoretical Foundations see below)

Nutrition: In terms of nutrition, we asked you first to get your calories in order. Then, we moved on to address protein daily needs and the accompanying tactics. This week, we focus on FIBER.

Get at least 40 grams a day, with a solid 20 in the nightly "fiber bomb". Fiber rushes things through your system. In fact, if you eat too much, it can prevent your body from absorbing all the energy (calories) from your food. This could be alarming if you are on the brink of starvation or severely malnourished, but it is not a terrible thing when dieting. Fiber will be your friend in your diet, along with protein and veggies. Your body doesn't digest it well, which means you feel full from it, but it doesn't add many calories to your total intake.

Habit: The new habit for this week is a "fiber bomb" before bed. This is a 20 gram-plus serving of fiber as your last snack (feel free to add protein if you need another protein feeding). It serves to push everything through your system, clean you out, keep you full, and more. If you hate going to bed hungry (me!), then you will appreciate this very much when we really get low on calories to push the weight-loss process.

For further information, we have videos on YouTube on fiber bomb suggestions. Search for "Fiber" on our YouTube Channel, "15minute.fitness".

Hydration: Also, this week we add 1 gallon of fluid per day. The research agrees that dehydration impairs fat loss through multiple mechanisms, and studies show most of the population is chronically dehydrated, so getting enough fluid is our next box to check. All fluid counts! Water is great because it is the best for flushing the kidneys, but all fluid counts in terms of hydration, and that is our present goal.

We personally love sugar-free drink packets. They are easy and come in so many flavors you are bound to find something you like! I also enjoy a big glass of tea that I brew daily. It contains green tea and oolong tea that have been shown to give a slight increase in metabolism. And, the caffeine is an energy boost. It also contains lemon that is good for your kidneys and ginger root that is good for bloat and digestion.

Jackie's Tea:
Brew in 2 quarts of very hot water or in tea maker
2 bags of green tea
2 bags of oolong tea
1 lemon, sliced
About 1 tablespoon sliced or diced fresh ginger root.

When I am done brewing, I add a 2qt size packet of sugar-free raspberry lemonade mix. You can add any flavor sugar-free drink mix you like, or you can add Splenda, or you can it drink as it is!

Weekly Challenge 4: Fiber & Hydration

1. Get over 40 grams of fiber per day total
2. Eat/Drink a "Fiber Bomb" before bed
3. Drink a gallon of fluid every day

CHAPTER 6
PHASE 2—DIET KICKSTART

Phase 2 is where we really start the diet proper. The goal is simple: to shift gears from muscle building and toning to emphasizing fat burning. Sometimes it takes a week or two (or three!) to push your body into fat burning mode. We have four weeks in this phase, so that's plenty of time to get the fire burning.

WEEK 5
MYO-REPS

Calorie Setup:

Overeaters & Maintainers: Did you hit a new low weight during this last week that was at least one pound lower than your low weight from the week before? If the answer is yes, then leave your calories the same this week. If the answer is no, then reduce your calories by 150 for a woman or 200 for a man. Remember, never reduce your calories below 800 for a woman or 1000 for a man under any circumstances. You will continue this feedback loop until Week Ten.

Undereaters: (Simple version) Drop your target calories by 400 calories for a woman and 700 calories for a man. You have now moved into Phase 2 of the diet.

(Complex version) Choose how aggressive you want to be on this diet. You can lose the same amount of weight in two different ways. You can reduce calories moderately over the course of 12 weeks or you can reduce calories more aggressively over the course of 6 to 8 weeks. This comes down to personal choice. Everyone's body responds slightly differently to moderate versus aggressive caloric reductions. And everyone has psychological preferences in terms of how long and how hard they want to diet. But, both methods usually result in very similar outcomes. Choose one now according to the numbers below.

Reduce your maintenance calorie total by 500 to 1000 calories depending on your choice above. Reduce it by 500 or so if you prefer a longer, milder diet. And reduce it by up to 1000 if you prefer a shorter, more aggressive diet. That said, there are a couple of more considerations to make before you choose your calorie deficit.

Because I never want a female below 800 calories or a male below 1200 calories, you have a built-in minimum number of calories. And because phase two of this program includes a feedback loop where you will continue to cut calories if your weight doesn't drop a certain amount each week, we can't get too close to our basement level calories just yet. Therefore, when you select your initial 500 to 1000 calorie drop, make sure your target number is not less than 1700 for a man or 1200 for a woman. That leaves us a little room for further tweaks later on throughout the 12-week program.

Challenge:
Exercise—Myo-Reps
(Theoretical Foundations p.56)

Training: This week begins our second, 4-week training block. We will deploy a new technique called Myo-Reps, allowing us to do more work in less time. More work in the same (or less) time is progression by VOLUME and DENSITY. That means more volume, more muscle-building stimulus and more calories going where we want them to go (muscle not fat).

There is an in-depth discussion of Myo-Reps in the section called Progression in the first Part of this book.

For further information, we have videos on YouTube demonstrating Myo-Reps. Search for "Myo-Reps" on our YouTube Channel, "15minute.fitness".

Weekly Challenge 5: Myo-Reps

Get familiar with this new training modality in your 6 workouts this week.

WEEK 6
MICRONUTRIENTS

Calorie Setup:

(ALL) Overeaters, Maintainers and Undereaters: did you hit a new low weight during this last week that was at least one pound lower than the lowest weight you hit the week before? If the answer is yes, then leave your calories the same this week. If the answer is no, then reduce your calories by 150 for a woman or 200 for a man. Remember, don't reduce your calories below 800 for a woman or 1200 for a man under any circumstances.

If you are at 800 (for a woman) or 1200 (for a man), and you do not hit a new low for 2 straight weeks, you need a longer metabolic priming phase—a complete Metabolic Reboot. Eat at maintenance for 8 straight weeks, and then begin again at week 1. If you have already done this (a full 8-week Metabolic Reboot), and this is your second time through, and you are still not able to lose weight, I would advise you to see a doctor and have a full metabolic panel of bloodwork done. You are likely deficient in output of a key hormone such as thyroid hormone (or thyroid-stimulating hormone—TSH).

Challenge:
Nutrition—Micronutrients
(Theoretical Foundations see below)

Micronutrients: We're still tracking calories, getting at least 4 solid protein meals each day and consuming 40g of fiber daily. Now we are drilling down to micronutrients—vitamins and minerals. We want you to log your food without any multivitamins you might be taking. Artificial sources of micros are ok, but natural food sources are better. And, vitamin & mineral rich foods form the foundation of a healthy and sustainable diet. This is a hard exercise—but it is enlightening to see the nutritional quality of the food you eat.

Keep TAKING your vitamin supplement, but DON'T LOG it in Cronometer.

For further information, please check out the charts in your "Resources" folder on your Member Dashboard (where you downloaded this book—just go to www.15minute.fitness and click "Member Login"). There, you'll find some healthy food suggestions to help you reach your micronutrient targets.

Weekly Challenge 6: Micronutrients

Try and turn your bars green in Cronometer using only real food choices.

(For those not using Cronometer [why not, there is a free version!], try and get 100% of your RDA requirements for all vitamins and minerals using natural foods alone)

WEEK 7
PRE-PLAN BREAKFAST

Calorie Setup:

(ALL) Overeaters, Maintainers and Undereaters: did you hit a new low weight during this last week that was at least one pound lower than the lowest weight you hit the week before? If the answer is yes, then leave your calories the same this week. If the answer is no, then reduce your calories by 150 for a woman or 200 for a man. Remember, don't reduce your calories below 800 for a woman or 1200 for a man under any circumstances.

If you are at 800 (for a woman) or 1200 (for a man), and you do not hit a new low for 2 straight weeks, you need a longer metabolic priming phase—a complete Metabolic Reboot. Eat at maintenance for 8 straight weeks, and then begin again at week 1. If you have already done this (a full 8-week Metabolic Reboot), and this is your second time through, and you are still not able to lose weight, I would advise you to see a doctor and have a full metabolic panel of bloodwork done. You are likely deficient in output of a key hormone such as thyroid hormone (or thyroid-stimulating hormone—TSH).

Challenge:
Nutrition—Meal Prep Breakfast
(Theoretical Foundations see below)

The key to consistent healthy eating is to have a plan. If you do not already know what you are going to eat for breakfast, then you will automatically lean toward convenience. Most pre-made, convenient breakfasts are full of sugars or starchy carbs, which set off your insulin response first thing in the morning. This makes you tired instead of energized (we mentioned this last week as a reason to eat carbs before bedtime!). It also predisposes your body to preferentially run on carbs rather than fat.

This week we want you to plan your breakfast for the entire week. This can be something you batch cook on Sunday and grab and go each morning (like an egg bake casserole) or something you have set out and can prepare quickly in the morning (like a smoothie or a wrap).

Look for ways to add vegetables to this meal—think spinach & mushroom omelet or spinach blended into your smoothies (really, you will not taste it) or grated zucchini in protein pancakes. (Grated zucchini cooked into pancakes tastes like carrot cake--don't ask me why.)

You can also eat like the Europeans. Breakfast in many parts of Europe is more like our lunch—sandwiches and wraps. Leftover stir fry also makes a good, healthy breakfast and is delicious mixed into scrambled eggs! Also, plan for "losing your plan." Maybe you woke up late or didn't get everything completely prepped the night before. Have a backup stash such as pre-made protein shakes or protein bars for mornings like this!

Unless you work out first thing in the morning, DO NOT eat starchy carbs or sugars for breakfast. Studies have found that your body will preferentially run on what you eat at your first meal of the day. If your breakfast is high in fat then your body will use more fat for fuel throughout the day thus burning more fat. Eggs do well at checking that box. If you are a morning smoothie person you may try adding some healthy fats to your smoothie such as avocado, MCT oil, or walnuts or almonds. If you can get a good, healthy meal at breakfast and lunch, it gives you more leeway at dinnertime, which is usually very welcome and allows you to fit in with your family at dinner.

Weekly Challenge 7: Pre-Plan Breakfast

Pre-Plan your breakfast--or first meal of the day--that includes veggies.

Homework: Post a pic of your breakfast (or first meal of the day) that includes veggies in our Facebook Group: "Fit Families of Faith" or our Facebook Page: "15 Minute Fitness".

WEEK 8
MEAL PREP—ALL MEALS

Calorie Setup:

(ALL) Overeaters, Maintainers and Undereaters: did you hit a new low weight during this last week that was at least one pound lower than the lowest weight you hit the week before? If the answer is yes, then leave your calories the same this week. If the answer is no, then reduce your calories by 150 for a woman or 200 for a man. Remember, don't reduce your calories below 800 for a woman or 1200 for a man under any circumstances.

If you are at 800 (for a woman) or 1200 (for a man), and you do not hit a new low for 2 straight weeks, you need a longer metabolic priming phase—a complete Metabolic Reboot. Eat at maintenance for 8 straight weeks, and then begin again at week 1. If you have already done this (a full 8-week Metabolic Reboot), and this is your second time through, and you are still not able to lose weight, I would advise you to see a doctor and have a full metabolic panel of bloodwork done. You are likely deficient in output of a key hormone such as thyroid hormone (or thyroid-stimulating hormone—TSH).

Challenge:
Nutrition—Pre-Plan All Meals
(Theoretical Foundations see below)

You should have practice meal-prepping breakfast. We started that last week. Now, we want you to extend that to lunch, and especially, supper. We want you to really try and get your family on board this week—even if that is just for one meal.

Cooking separate meals for you and your kids is wrong on so many levels. First off, children need healthy food just like adults. Second, it sucks for you. That's double the meal prep, and if you prepare unhealthy versions of your dinner for your children, it is temptation right in your face to eat trash.

See if you can find one healthy meal you can all sit down and eat together. Snap a picture of it, and post it for all the other parents who are stuck in that same trap. It is an inspiration and a service to those who think they have no hope.

We really want to make some lasting lifestyle changes that affect your families for the better. We want families to have shared, healthy family-meals whenever possible. This strengthens your bodies, your children's bodies, and most importantly, your family unit. These are high-level life-goals here.

The focus for Phases two and three is fat loss. This is accomplished mainly through reducing calories while meeting protein, micronutrient (micros) and fiber needs. Adding lots of veggies to your meals helps you feel full and get your micros. If you are still struggling to add veggies in place of the starchy carbs and fats, then keep working on that and check out our recipe book for specific ideas. You can find that on our website www.15minute.fitness.

Weekly Challenge 8: Pre-Plan All Meals

1. Pre-Plan your dinners for the whole week

Homework: Post a pic of the meal the rest of your family most enjoys in our Facebook Group: "Fit Families of Faith" or our Facebook Page: "15 Minute Fitness".

CHAPTER 7
PHASE 3—DIET AFTERBURN

Phase 3 is where we pull out all the stops to keep the fat burning ball rolling as far and as fast as it will go. This is the end phase of the diet cycle. As calories drop lower, just remember, it is only for a couple more weeks. Then, you will cycle out, reboot your metabolism, eat some good food, build and tone some more muscle, and only then, start over again.

Let's squeeze what we can out of this cycle, though. Once you have momentum, do everything you can to keep it!

WEEK 9
7-DAY KETO CHALLENGE

Calorie Setup:

(ALL) Overeaters, Maintainers and Undereaters: did you hit a new low weight during this last week that was at least one pound lower than the lowest weight you hit the week before? If the answer is yes, then leave your calories the same this week. If the answer is no, then reduce your calories by 150 for a woman or 200 for a man. Remember, don't reduce your calories below 800 for a woman or 1200 for a man under any circumstances.

If you are at 800 (for a woman) or 1200 (for a man), and you do not hit a new low for 2 straight weeks, you need a longer metabolic priming phase—a complete Metabolic Reboot. Eat at maintenance for 8 straight weeks, and then begin again at week 1. If you have already done this (a full 8-week Metabolic Reboot), and this is your second time through, and you are still not able to lose weight, I would advise you to see a doctor and have a full metabolic panel of bloodwork done. You are likely deficient in output of a key hormone such as thyroid hormone (or thyroid-stimulating hormone—TSH).

Challenge:
Nutrition—7-Day Keto Challenge
(Theoretical Foundations see below)

Our overall target for the twelve weeks is to shed around 10% of your body weight in body fat. That number/percentage may be confounded if you are simultaneously gaining muscle while losing fat, but then you will be losing pant sizes and looking more awesome in front of a mirror, so weight won't matter.

You are all on a low-calorie, high-protein diet model. As such, there has not been much room for carbs under your calorie cap. I want to kick off the final 4 week block with a 7-day keto challenge, where you squeeze out those last few remaining carbs. For guys, this means less than 40 "net carbs" per day ("net carbs", for us, means total carbohydrates minus fiber). For ladies, this means less than 30 net carbs per day.

This will put you into ketosis. While there is no special magic to ketosis (and in my opinion, long-term ketogenic diets are not the best (for many reasons including health, performance and quality of life), ketosis is a useful tool to hasten fat-loss when it slows, and to restart fat-loss when you stall out.

If you look through your Cronometer, I'll bet you can find some places you can chop away some carbs on a daily basis. I'm not asking you to do this forever—just one week. If you see your weight loss speeding up, we might want to extend that. If not, we put that tool back in the bag and try another.

Warning: Keto is stricter than what we have been doing on the Sine-Wave Diet. With the Sine-Wave, you have flexibility—if you eat too many calories one day, you make up in the next day or two. It doesn't work that way with carbs and ketosis. Once you're in ketosis (it takes about 3 days at very low carb levels to enter ketosis), a single high carb day kicks you out of ketosis—far less flexible and forgiving. Try it for a week.

Weekly Challenge 9: Keto Challenge

1. Set Cronometer to track "net carbs" in your settings, and cut your net carbs down to less than 40 grams per day (for a man) or 30 grams per day (for a woman).

WEEK 10
INTENTIONAL ACTIVITY

Calorie Setup:

(ALL) Overeaters, Maintainers and Undereaters: did you hit a new low weight during this last week that was at least one pound lower than the lowest weight you hit the week before? If the answer is yes, then leave your calories the same this week. If the answer is no, then reduce your calories by 150 for a woman or 200 for a man. Remember, don't reduce your calories below 800 for a woman or 1200 for a man under any circumstances.

If you are at 800 (for a woman) or 1200 (for a man), and you do not hit a new low for 2 straight weeks, you need a longer metabolic priming phase—a complete Metabolic Reboot. Eat at maintenance for 8 straight weeks, and then begin again at week 1. If you have already done this (a full 8-week Metabolic Reboot), and this is your second time through, and you are still not able to lose weight, I would advise you to see a doctor and have a full metabolic panel of bloodwork done. You are likely deficient in output of a key hormone such as thyroid hormone (or thyroid-stimulating hormone—TSH).

Challenge:
Exercise—Intentional Activity
(Theoretical Foundations see below)

You know I am not a big fan of cardio for the purposes of body composition change. Your caloric expenditure from daily activity is a MUCH smaller part of your total daily caloric expenditure than is your Resting Metabolic Rate (RMR). And that (RMR) is what we are boosting over the long term by adding muscle.

That said, there is a time and a season when expending extra calories through activity makes sense—and that time is now.

When you are deep into a diet, your body looks for every imaginable way to conserve energy. So, consciously adding in activity can mitigate that metabolic slowdown from your body trying to preserve itself from starvation. This phenomenon of metabolic adaptation to diets is why you eventually plateau in any diet and have to cycle out and reboot your metabolism before going for another round of successful dieting.

Also, when you are deep into a diet, the balance of the calorie expenditure equation shifts a bit. Here's what I mean. Say jogging on a treadmill for an hour burns 200 calories (for example only—everyone will spend a different amount of calories doing any activity). When you are taking in 2000 calories a day, that's not a huge deal. Whoopee—an hour of my life gone forever to sweat-inducing drudgery for an extra 10% calorie burn. That's a bad trade-off in my view.

But, when your daily budget of calories gets down to 1000, the trade-off becomes a bit more tempting—that same hour is now worth an extra 20% calorie burn.

Does this mean I want you to roll out of bed and slog away on the treadmill? No. "Activity" encompasses FAR MORE than mind-numbing cardio. Think "productive activity". Do the dishes. Mow the lawn. Walk the dog. Do yardwork. Do laundry. All activity counts, and I'd much rather see you playing with your kids or knocking out chores and honey-do's than wasting your time on a cardio machine.

"But I work all week!" I get it. Try doing it on the weekend. Some is better than none—it's not an all-or-nothing thing. And ideally, these should be productive, life-enhancing activities—things you need, or have been wanting, to do anyway. Now you have extra motivation to do them. They will help your fat come off faster right now while you are deep into your diet.

During these last 3 weeks, ANY bit of extra activity you can force yourself to do will be helpful in combatting the body's natural tendency to conserve energy during periods of low energy intake (metabolic adaptation to dieting).

Additionally, there is some mixed evidence in the scientific literature for an extra fat burning benefit from "fasted activity" vs "fed activity". So, you might intentionally do something before you have your first meal. This probably makes only a very small difference, but everyone wants to know "optimum"—there it is.

Weekly Challenge 10: Intentional Activity

1. Consciously add some activities, chores, projects and honey-do's to keep your metabolism up and boost your total daily caloric expenditure, especially before your first meal.

Homework: Make a post to share what you did in our Facebook Group: "Fit Families of Faith" or our Facebook Page: "15 Minute Fitness".

WEEK 11
PROTEIN SPARING MODIFIED FAST
(PSMF)

Calorie Setup:

NEW (ALL) Overeaters, Maintainers and Undereaters: For the next two weeks (2 weeks ONLY), there is no minimum calorie level. See below.

Challenge:
Nutrition—Protein Sparing Modified Fast
(Theoretical Foundations see below)

Phase 3 is where we kick weight loss into high gear. Phase 1 revved your metabolism. Phase 2 got the ball rolling, and phase 3 is where we pull out all the stops to wash off body fat as fast and as far as possible.

Let's test your creativity. For the last 2 weeks of the diet, as long as you meet your protein, fiber and micronutrient requirements, you may go as low as you like in calories.

There is such a thing as a Protein-Sparing Modified Fast (PSMF). This is essentially protein, green veggies, vitamin supplements...and nothing else. It is prescribed for the clinical treatment of obesity by doctors in metabolic wards.

You are very near PSMF conditions already. This is your opportunity to be ruthless in rooting out every last unnecessary calorie in your diet. This is not where I want you to "live" for long. This is only these last two weeks. Then, we'll re-assess and break from dieting for a bit.

For the next 2 weeks, there IS NO MINIMUM calorie requirement. YOU may go as low as you like as long as you meet your protein, fiber and micronutrient requirements. Look at every single calorie you put in your mouth. Does it contribute to protein? Does it help meet your fiber target? Is it full of micronutrients? If not, leave it. Most veggies are nearly void of calories, so I want you to keep them in for the natural micros they provide. Make sure you are taking a full-spectrum multivitamin too!

JONAS & JACKIE SCHWARTZ

Weekly Challenge 11: Protein-Sparing Modified Fast

See how low you can drop calories while still meeting protein, fiber and micronutrient goals.

WEEK 12
REVERSE DIETING & FUTURE
PLANNING

Challenge:
Nutrition—Reverse Dieting
(Theoretical Foundations see below)

At this point, we are most interested in figuring out
when to come out of the diet phase. There are basically
two factors to consider when making this choice.

1.   Physiological: Your body has ceased to make
changes. Your scale weight is not dropping anymore,
an/or you don't notice continuing differences in the
way your clothes fit. Our coaching decisions usually
revolve around scale-weight, because that is the most
readily accessible data we have before us. So, my rule of
thumb is this: if you go to full weeks without a new low,
it's time to pull the plug and begin reverse diet.

2.   Psychological: your mind is just "done" with
living on a low-calorie diet. Maybe you are having food

fantasies all the time, even dreaming about food. Maybe you are grouchy, depressed, or miserably low on energy. These are legitimate reasons for halting the diet and beginning to climb back up slowly to maintenance in order to take a break.

Okay, once you have decided enough is enough and you are ready for a break, what then? In general, we want to bring you up to maintenance level calories as fast as possible without you regaining body fat. You can expect to regain a couple of pounds in the first week when you reintroduce carbs, because they will cause you to store more water in your muscle tissue. So, your muscles are going to swell. The scale won't like you, but the mirror definitely will.

All right, so what kind of guidelines can I give that are general enough to apply to everyone? Keep in mind, each individual is different, so the rate at which we can reintroduce calories will differ with every particular body. That said, if I was forced to write an algorithm to describe my decision-making process as your coach during the reverse diet, it would be along the lines of the following:

1. Estimate your new maintenance calorie level. You can do this in Cronometer. That will be our target. We need to get up there slowly though so as not to regain fat.

2. Find the difference between your present calorie level and that maintenance calorie level (maintenance calorie target - present calorie intake). Add 50% of that back this week and the remaining balance the next week.

Admittedly, that's an oversimplification. and I would

want to watch your weight over that first week to determine whether that was too many or too few calories. And the same the following week. But, that's a general guideline.

I'd like you to hold your new maintenance for 4 weeks at a minimum before attempting another 8-week diet. Your metabolism right now is very sluggish because you have been starving yourself for the past couple of months. It needs some time to heal and get revved back up. The longer you give it to heal, the easier your next diet phase will be.

Now, during your maintenance phase, I would continue to try to bump up your calories little by little as high as possible without the scale running away on you. I cannot tell you what that number is for you as an individual. If you attempt this on your own, try adding 100 or 150 calories and see if your weight noticeably jumps during the week. (I would expect about a half-pound to a pound per week average weight-gain during this phase.) If you are working out hard, this should be largely muscle gain. That's what we want.

if your weight does not move up, do it again—add another 100-150 calories. Do this until your weight does jump up a couple pounds, and then back off 50 or 100 calories. Hold that level for a while. The higher you can boost your maintenance-level calories, the easier and more effective the next diet phase will be for you. (Metabolic adaptation works both ways—you can actually slowly train your body to maintain on higher calorie levels—just like it learned to subsist on low calorie levels.)

If you are going to program your own workouts, just repeat what we've done during this program (see

Appendix A for a sample). Those are fundamentally sound workouts that hit every major muscle group in your body multiple times per week. You are now eating a good bit of calories, so you can challenge yourself a little bit more during those workouts. Try to add a rep here and there; try to add a set here and there; and even try to bump your weights up slowly over time. (See the section on "Progression" in the first part of the book.) Don't do anything radical. Slow and steady progress wins this race. The last thing you want is an injury.

After you have completed a 4 week maintenance (muscle-building) cycle, you may repeat these 12 weekly challenges to lose more fat. Rotate the 12 week diet with the 4 week maintenance over and over until you are at your goal body composition. It really is that simple!

AFTERWORD

I sincerely hope you have learned a new perspective on achieving lifetime health, strength and leanness from this book. I know some of the parts might have been hard to follow, but all of our clients, after going through the 12 week program get the experiential understanding of how to make this structure work easily and simply in their particular lives.

It is hard writing for a very general audience. An author has to balance the simplicity of necessary general principles with the complexity of the myriad ways those principles might apply to specific individuals with specific circumstances, specific needs, specific constraints, etc. Absolutely everything you need in order to change your body for good is within these pages, but I will definitely invite anyone who wishes to be guided through the process (at least once) to try out our premium program. I believe it offers THE MOST comprehensive value in terms of lifetime learning and right-now results of any program available anywhere. It always helps to be led through difficult terrain by a guide before setting oof on one's own.

Whether you take that path or not, I exhort you to give this program a real try. Everyone who gives it a sincere try gets amazing results and reports back that it is FAR easier than they had been led to believe. We live in an era of scientific research and wide dissemination of information. There is no more reason for radical diets which cut out entire categories of foods as taboo. There is no more reason to spend an hour in the gym killing your soul with cardio or putting yourself in mortal danger for permanent injury throwing around weights in unstable positions. There is a better way. We at 15 Minute Fitness want to bring enlightened, evidence-based health and fitness principles to real people with real families and real lives. Our prayer is that we help families break the generational curse of obesity and disease. We hope you will join the movement.

Blessings!
Jonas & Jackie Schwartz

P.S. If you feel like anything in this book has benefitted you in any way, we would really appreciate you taking a second and leaving a review on Amazon. We really want this message to spread in order to help others who are overwhelmed and lost. Thank you!

CONTACT US

Feel free to reach out to us. We'd love to hear from you!

www.15minute.fitness (website)
Fit Families of Faith (FB Group)
15 Minute Fitness (FB Page)
support@15minute.fitness (email)

APPENDIX A

SAMPLE WORKOUT ROUTINE

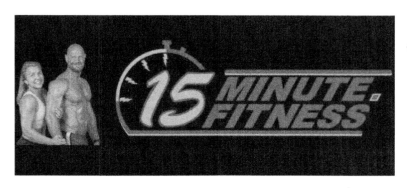

Your First Month
Beginner Workout (At Home)

Day	Workout	Exercise	Sets[1]	Reps[2]	Weight[3]	Rest
Monday/Thursday	Push		1-4	20-30		60
		Pushups			Body	seconds
		Overhead Press	1-4	5-30		60 seconds
Tuesday/Friday						60
	Pull	Bent Over Rows	1-4	20-30		seconds
		Upright Rows	1-4	5-30		60 seconds
Wednesday/Saturday		Sumo Squats	1-4	20-30		60 seconds
	Legs					
		Stiff Legged Sumo Deadlifts	1-4	5-30		60 seconds

[1] SETS—1st week do one set each. 2nd week do 2 sets. 3rd week do 3 sets. 4th week do 4 sets. Now you are ready to progress to a full-on program.

[2] REPS   First exercise in each workout: 20-30 reps. 2nd exercise: 5-30 reps (choose weight accordingly)

[3] WEIGHT   Select a weight that allows you to perform 20-30 reps (1st exercise) and 5-30 reps (2nd exercise). If you cannot perform the minimum number of reps within range, your weight is too heavy. If you can perform more than 30 reps, your weight is too light.

Moving Forward

If you bought a copy of this book, then I will give you 30 day access to my free beginner's workout program on the training app we use with our paid clients, "15minute.fitness". Just go to www.15minute.fitness and sign up for our "Free Foundations Course." It is a 1 page course with short videos that explains our basic approach. At the end of that page, you'll find the offer for free app access.

Too many people fail in their health and fitness pursuits due to lack of preparation. Taking the little time necessary to lay solid foundations makes all the difference. Our clients who have followed that 1 page course have shown exponentially better results than those who choose not to.

If you would like our ready-made 12 week course that walks you through this program one week at a time (both diet and weekly progressive workout routines), please check out our Premium program on www.15minute.fitness.

We also offer an Essentials (workouts-only) program which guides you through progressive 15 minute daily workouts. It insures you continue to provide the necessary level of stimulus required to keep your progress moving ever forward.

You have all the tools you need. All you have to do now is put it into practice! If you need further help implementing this, we're always here for you!

Blessings!

t

Printed in Great Britain
by Amazon

68966263R00098